Dosage Calculations

an

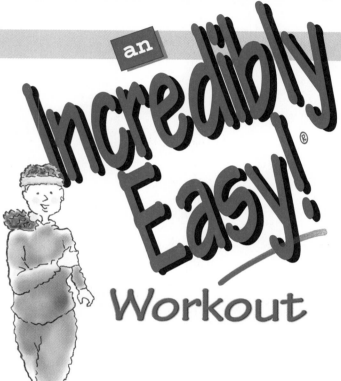

Incredibly Easy!®

Workout

Dosage Calculations

an Incredibly Easy! Workout

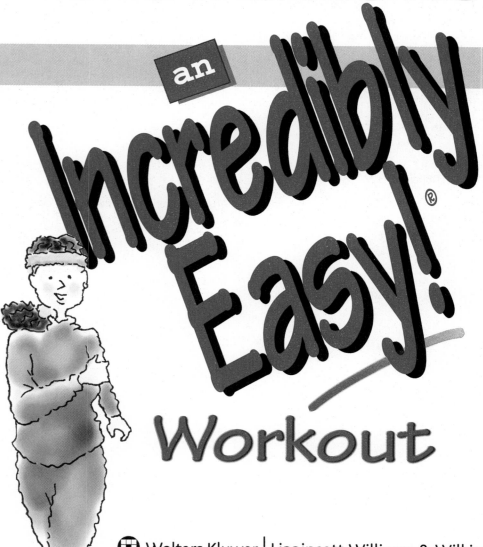

Wolters Kluwer | Lippincott Williams & Wilkins
Health

Philadelphia · Baltimore · New York · London
Buenos Aires · Hong Kong · Sydney · Tokyo

Staff

Executive Publisher
Judith A. Schilling McCann, RN, MSN

Editorial Director
David Moreau

Clinical Director
Joan M. Robinson, RN, MSN

Art Director
Mary Ludwicki

Editorial Project Manager
Gabrielle Mosquera

Clinical Project Manager
Jennifer Meyering, RN, BSN, MS, CCRN

Editors
Karen C. Comerford, Maureen M. Salera, Susan Williams

Copy Editors
Kimberly Bilotta (supervisor), Jeannine Fielding,
Dorothy P. Terry, Pamela Wingrod

Designers
Lynn Foulk, Georg W. Purvis IV

Illustrator
Bot Roda

Digital Composition Services
Diane Paluba (manager), Joyce R. Biletz, Donald Knauss,
Donna S. Morris

Associate Manufacturing Manager
Beth J. Welsh

Editorial Assistants
Karen J. Kirk, Jeri O'Shea, Linda K. Ruhf

Workout regimen

1 Math basics 1

2 Measurement systems 31

3 Recording drug administration 43

4 Oral, topical, and rectal drugs 67

5 Calculating parenteral injections 101

6 Calculating I.V. infusions 133

7 Special calculations 173

Answers 206

1

Math basics

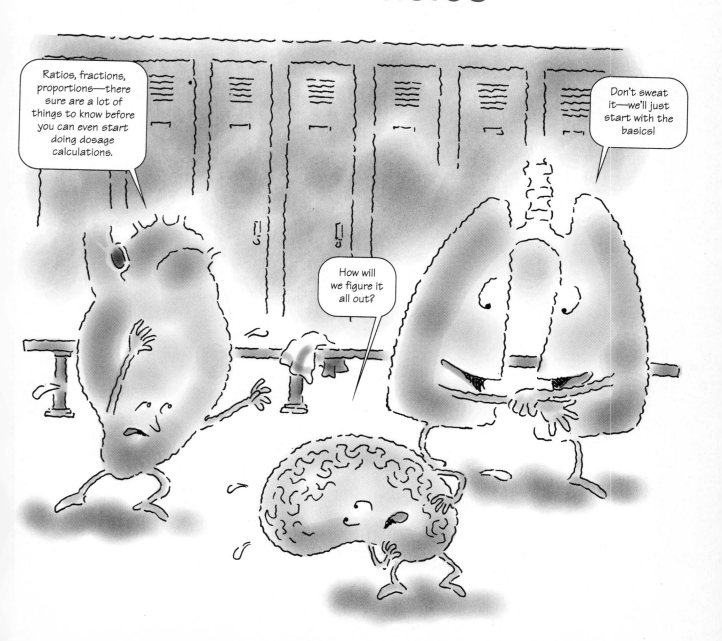

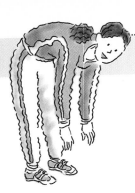

Math basics review

Fraction basics

- A fraction is a mathematical expression for parts of a whole.
- The denominator (bottom number) represents the total number of equal parts in the whole.
- The numerator (top number) represents the number of parts of the whole being considered.

Reducing fractions

- Determine the largest common divisor.
- Divide the numerator and denominator by that number.

Common denominators

- Multiply all the denominators in a set of fractions to find the common denominator.
- The smallest multiple of the denominators is the lowest common denominator.

Adding and subtracting fractions

- Always convert to fractions with common denominators first, then add or subtract the numerators and keep the denominator as it is.

Multiplying fractions

- Multiply the numerators and denominators in turn.

Dividing fractions

- Write them as two fractions separated by a division sign.
- Invert the divisor.
- Multiply the dividend by the inverted divisor.

Decimals and percentages

- A decimal fraction is a proper fraction in which the denominator is a power of 10, signified by a decimal point placed at the left of the numerator.
- A percentage is any quantity stated as parts per hundred (the percent sign takes the place of the denominator 100).

Multiplying decimals

- The number of decimal places in the product equals the sum of the decimal places in the numbers multiplied.

Dividing decimals

- When a whole number is the divisor, place the quotient's decimal point directly above the dividend's decimal point.
- When a decimal fraction is the divisor, move the divisor's decimal point to the right to convert to a whole number, then move the dividend's decimal the same number of places to the right and, lastly, place the quotient's decimal point directly above the dividend's decimal point.

Rounding off decimals

- Check the number to the right of the decimal place that will be rounded off.
- If that number is less than 5, leave the number in the decimal place alone and delete the number less than 5.
- If that number is 5 or greater, add 1 to the decimal place and delete the number greater than 5.

Converting percentages to decimals

- Multiply the percentage number by $\frac{1}{100}$ (or 0.01).
- Or, shift the decimal two places to the left.

Converting decimals to percentages

- Divide the decimal fraction by $\frac{1}{100}$ (or 0.01).
- Or, shift the decimal two places to the right.

Converting percentages to common fractions

- Remove the percent sign.
- Move the decimal point two places to the left.
- Convert to a common fraction with a denominator that's a factor of 10.

Finding a percentage of a number

- Restate as a multiplication problem by changing the word *of* to a multiplication sign.
- Convert the percentage to a decimal fraction.
- Multiply the two numbers.

Finding what percentage one number is of another

- Restate as a division problem.
- Convert the quotient to a percentage.
- If there's a remainder from the division problem, state the quotient as a mixed number by turning the remainder into a common fraction.

Finding a number when you know a percentage of it

- Convert the percentage into a decimal fraction.
- Divide the number by the decimal fraction.

Numerical relationship basics

- *Ratio:* uses a colon between the numbers in a numerical relationship
- *Fraction:* uses a slash between numbers in a numerical relationship
- *Proportion:* a statement of equality between two ratios or two fractions

Solving common-fraction equations

- Multiply numerators.
- Multiply denominators.
- Restate the equation.
- Reduce the fraction.
- Convert the fraction to decimal form by dividing the numerator by the denominator.

Solving decimal-fraction equations

- Move the decimal points two spaces to the right.
- Remove the zeros.
- Convert the whole number to a fraction.
- Multiply the numerators.
- Multiply the denominators.
- Restate the equation.
- Convert the answer to a decimal form by dividing the numerator by the denominator.

Solving proportions with ratios

- Means—middle numbers
- Extremes—end numbers
- Product of the means = product of the extremes
- Isolate X on one side of the equation.
- Solve for X.

Solving proportions with fractions

- Cross products of a proportion are always equal.
- Multiply the cross products.
- Put the cross products into the equation, and isolate X on one side of the equation.
- Solve for X.

Dimensional analysis basics

- Use whenever two quantities are directly proportional to each other.
- Use common equivalents or conversion factors to convert to the same unit of measurement.
- Set up the problem using fractions.

Performing dimensional analysis—6 steps

- Determine the given quantity.
- Determine the wanted quantity.
- Select conversion factors.
- Set up the problem.
- Cancel unwanted units.
- Multiply the numerators, multiply the denominators, and divide the products.

■■ ■ Finish line

Label the numerator and denominator in each of these fractions.

1. _____ $\dfrac{2}{3}$

2. _____

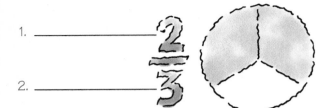

3. _____ $\dfrac{5}{16}$

4. _____

■■ ■ Match point

Match each fraction to its type.

Clues

1. Common _____

2. Complex _____

3. Proper _____

4. Improper _____

Options

A. $\dfrac{1}{4}$

B. $\dfrac{5/6}{3/4}$

C. $\dfrac{2}{3}$

D. $\dfrac{9}{5}$

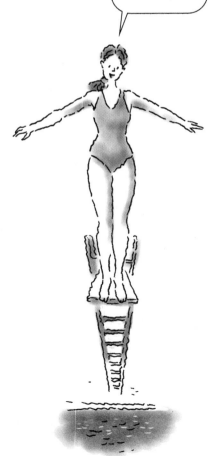

Watch me dive right into these basics!

■ Hit or miss

Label each statement with a "T" for "True" or an "F" for "False."

_____ 1. You can manipulate fractions by finding a common numerator.

_____ 2. The mixed number $2\frac{1}{5}$ converted to an improper fraction is $\frac{11}{5}$.

_____ 3. A fraction should usually be reduced to its lowest terms.

_____ 4. The fraction $\frac{3}{10}$ can be reduced further.

_____ 5. Multiplying all of the denominators in a set of fractions will give you a common denominator.

■ Finish line

Each pie chart shows a fraction of a pie. Label each pie with the correct fraction.

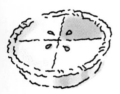
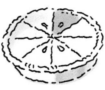
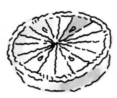
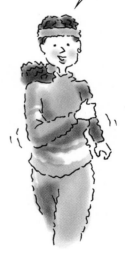

1. _____   2. _____   3. _____

■■ ■ Finish line

Fill in each blank decimal place with its power of 10.

1. _____

2. _____

3. _____

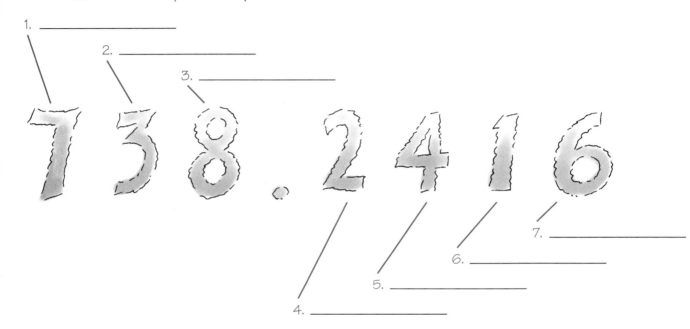

4. _____

5. _____

6. _____

7. _____

■■ ■ Strikeout

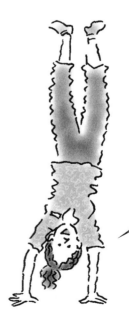

Don't give up—
all this effort will
add up in the end!

Strike out the decimal fractions that have been rounded off incorrectly.

Original fractions	Rounded fractions
1. 5.346	5.34
2. 10.592	10.59
3. 4.666	4.67
4. 7.324	7.33
5. 15.014	15.02

Batter's box

Fill in the blanks of this decimal fact with the correct information regarding fractions.

To change a percent to a decimal fraction, remove the _____ sign and

1

_____ the number in the percentage by _____ or 0.01.

2   3

Options

A. multiply

B. $\dfrac{1}{100}$

C. percent

Starting lineup

Put these steps in the order needed to convert $\frac{1}{3}$ into a decimal.

Divide 1 by 3	
Round to 0.33	
Take $\frac{1}{3}$	
Take 0.333	

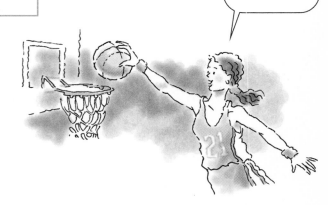

Solving this one should be a slam dunk!

■ Match point

Match the numerical relationship with its correct name.

Clues

1. 3 : 4 _____
2. ¾ _____
3. 3 : 4 :: 6 : 8 _____

Options

A. Proportion
B. Ratio
C. Fraction

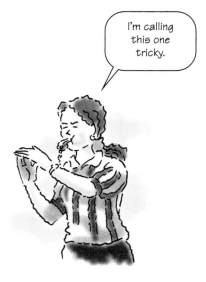

■ You make the call

Fill in the correct answer.

Question: If the hospital workout room has 10 stationary bikes, and three nurses want to use them, what is the relationship of nurses to bikes?

Answer: _____

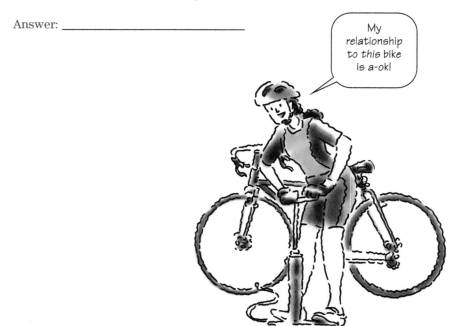

Hit or miss

Is this statement true or false? Label it with a "T" for "True" or an "F" for "False."

Question: If it takes one nurse to lift 2 lbs of medical supplies, then it takes eight nurses to lift 24 lbs of medical supplies.

Answer: _____

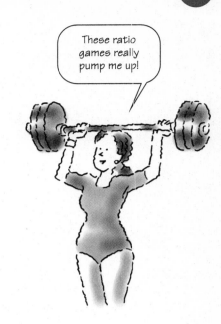

Strikeout

Strike out the incorrect equation.

$$\frac{100 \text{ syringes}}{1 \text{ box}} = \frac{200 \text{ syringes}}{2 \text{ boxes}}$$

$$\frac{200 \text{ beds}}{1 \text{ hospital}} = \frac{600 \text{ beds}}{3 \text{ hospitals}}$$

$$\frac{150 \text{ bedpans}}{1 \text{ floor}} = \frac{325 \text{ bedpans}}{3 \text{ floors}}$$

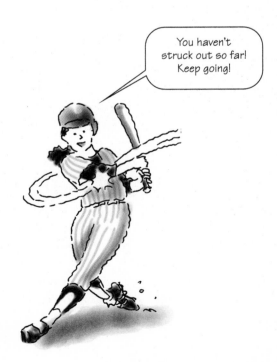

■ ■
■ Jumble gym

Unscramble the underlined letters to form the answer to the question.

Question: What term is commonly used to describe a person or event that could cause unexpected or unknown outcomes?

Daily exercise promotes a healthy outlook.
Exercise can also be fun.
Try to get out and about a few times a week.

Answer: __ __ __ __ __ __ __

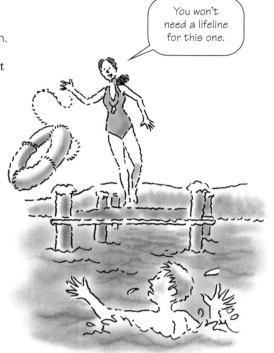

You won't need a lifeline for this one.

■ ■
■ Batter's box

Fill in the blanks with the correct information regarding proportions.

The unknown ratio or fraction in a proportion is represented by _____ . You
                                                                          1
can solve for X to determine the _____ of the _____ quantity.
                                              2   3

Options

A. value

B. unknown

C. X

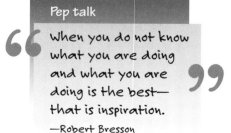

Pep talk

When you do not know what you are doing and what you are doing is the best— that is inspiration.

—Robert Bresson

■■
■ Starting lineup

Part one: Five steps are needed to solve the equation $X = \frac{1}{5} \times \frac{3}{9}$. Place these worded steps in their proper order.

Multiply the denominators.	
Reduce the fraction.	
Multiply the numerators.	
Restate the equation.	
Convert the equation to decimal form.	

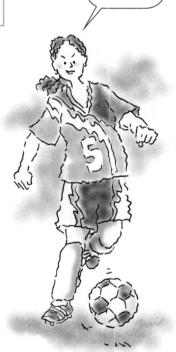

The goal here is to know your steps.

■■
■ Starting lineup

Part two: Now let's do the math and solve the same equation for X by putting these numerical steps in the proper order.

$X = \frac{1}{5} \times \frac{3}{9}$	
$X = \frac{3}{3} \div \frac{45}{3} = \frac{1}{15}$	
$1 \times 3 = 3$	
$X = \frac{1 \times 3}{5 \times 9} = \frac{3}{45}$	
$5 \times 9 = 45$	
$X = \frac{1}{15} = 1 \div 15 = 0.07$	

■ Batter's box

Fill in the blanks with the correct information regarding converting fractions.

To convert a fraction to a _____ , divide the _____ by the

               1   2

_____ . Round the _____ off to the nearest

     3   4

_____ .

    5

Options

A. denominator

B. hundredth

C. numerator

D. decimal

E. answer

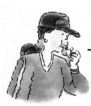

Coaching session

Explaining X

Being able to find the value of *X* is a critical skill for making dosage calculations. For example, if a doctor orders a drug for your patient but the drug isn't available in the ordered strength, it's up to you to figure out the right amount of drug to administer. Here's an example of how to do it.

Let's say you receive an order to administer 0.1 mg of epinephrine subcutaneously, but the only epinephrine available is a 1-ml ampule containing 1 mg of the drug. Start your calculation by stating the problem in a proportion:

    1 mg : 1 ml :: 0.1 mg : *X* ml

Rewrite the problem as an equation by applying the principle that the product of the means equals the product of the extremes.

    1 ml × 0.1 mg = 1 mg × *X* ml

Solve for *X* by dividing both sides of the equation by the known value that appears on the same side of the equation as the unknown value *X*. Then cancel out units that appear in the numerator and denominator, isolating *X* on one side of the equation.

$$\frac{1\ ml \times 0.1\ \cancel{mg}}{1\ \cancel{mg}} = \frac{1\ \cancel{mg} \times X\ ml}{1\ \cancel{mg}}$$

    X = 0.1 ml

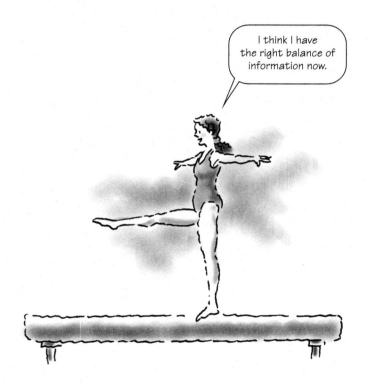

I think I have the right balance of information now.

██ You make the call

Time to tone up your knowledge of common-fraction equations! Which one of these examples gives you the correct answer?

1.

$$X = \frac{1}{6} \times \frac{4}{5}$$

$$X = \frac{1 \times 4}{6 \times 5} = \frac{4}{30}$$

$$X = 4 \div \frac{2}{30} \div 2 = \frac{2}{15}$$

2.

$$X = \frac{1}{6} \times \frac{4}{5}$$

$$X = \frac{1 \times 6}{5 \times 4} = \frac{6}{20}$$

$$X = 2 \div \frac{2}{20} \div 2 = \frac{3}{10}$$

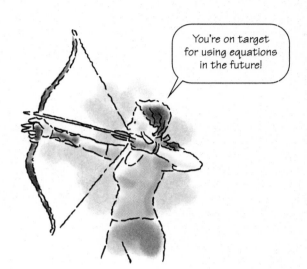

You're on target for using equations in the future!

██ Strikeout

Which decimal is correctly converted from the fraction in the correct answer in the game above? Strike out the incorrect decimals.

1. 0.25
2. 1.31
3. 0.13
4. 0.19
5. 0.46

■ Cross-training

Test your knowledge of fractions and decimals with this review.

Across

2. In a decimal number, the decimal separates the _____ number from the decimal fraction.

6. Type of fraction where the top number is bigger than the bottom number

8. In a decimal fraction, the bottom number is a power of _____ .

9. The top number in a fraction; represents the number of parts of the whole being considered

Down

1. The bottom number in a fraction; represents the total number of equal parts in the whole

3. Type of fraction; also a synonym for "elaborate"

4. A fraction represents the _____ of one number by another.

5. Type of fraction where the top number is smaller than the bottom number

7. Type of fraction; also the opposite of "rare"

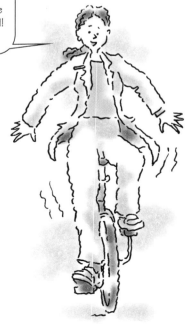

Your knowledge of this topic sure isn't fractional! Go get 'em!

Starting lineup

Four steps are needed to solve the equation $X = {}^{150}\!/_{600} \times 3$ as a decimal number. Place these steps in their proper order.

$X = \dfrac{450}{600}$	
$X = \dfrac{150}{600} \times \dfrac{3}{1}$	
$X = \dfrac{3}{4} = 3 \div 4 = 0.75$	
$X = \dfrac{150 \times 3}{600 \times 1}$	

Getting these equation steps down may be a hurdle, but it'll pay off later.

Match point

Match the equation with its correct answer.

Clues

1. $X = \dfrac{1}{3} \times \dfrac{3}{8}$ _____

2. $X = \dfrac{2}{5} \times \dfrac{3}{4}$ _____

3. $X = \dfrac{3}{4} \times \dfrac{3}{5}$ _____

4. $X = \dfrac{2}{7} \times \dfrac{5}{8}$ _____

5. $X = \dfrac{1}{4} \times \dfrac{2}{3}$ _____

Options

A. .45
B. .30
C. .17
D. .12
E. .18

■■ Batter's box

Fill in the blanks with the correct information regarding decimal fractions.

To solve for X in equations with decimal fractions, _____ the decimal
1

_____ from the fraction by moving them to the _____ . Then
2 3

remove the _____ . Next, convert the whole number to a _____ .
4 5

Multiply the _____ , then multiply the _____ .
6 7

Restate the equation. Convert the answer to _____ form.
8

Options

A. points

B. decimal

C. fraction

D. remove

E. zeros

F. denominators

G. right

H. numerators

■■ Starting lineup

Put these steps in the order needed to finish the calculation $X = {}^{0.25}\!/0.12 \times 0.5$.

$12 \times 1 = 12$

$X = \dfrac{25}{12} \times \dfrac{0.5}{1}$

$25 \times 0.5 = 12.5$

$X = \dfrac{12.5}{12} = 12.5 \div 12 = 1.04$

$X = \dfrac{25 \times 0.5}{12 \times 1} = \dfrac{12.5}{12}$

Pep talk

" The world looks like a multiplication table, or a mathematical equation, which, turn it how you will, balances itself. "

—Ralph Waldo Emerson

■ Match point

Match the equation with its correct decimal equivalent.

Clues

1. $\dfrac{8.2}{3}$ _____

2. $\dfrac{11.4}{4}$ _____

3. $\dfrac{10.2}{5}$ _____

4. $\dfrac{6.3}{1}$ _____

5. $\dfrac{2.7}{6}$ _____

Options

A. 2.85

B. 0.45

C. 2.7

D. 6.3

E. 2.04

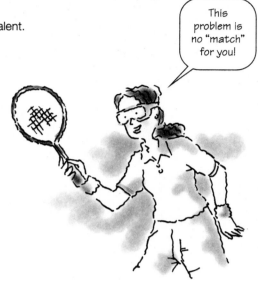

This problem is no "match" for you!

■ Hit or miss

Did we hit the mark and get the correct answer here? Label it with a "T" for "True" or an "F" for "False."

$$X = \frac{0.44}{0.12 \times 0.5}$$

$$X = \frac{44}{12} \times 0.5$$

$$X = \frac{44}{12} \times \frac{0.5}{1}$$

$$44 \times 0.5 = 2.20$$

$$12 \times 1 = 12$$

$$X = \frac{44 \times 0.5}{12 \times 1} = \frac{2.20}{12} = 0.28$$

Answer: _____

■ Finish line

Label the parts of this proportion.

1. _____

2. _____

3. _____

4. _____

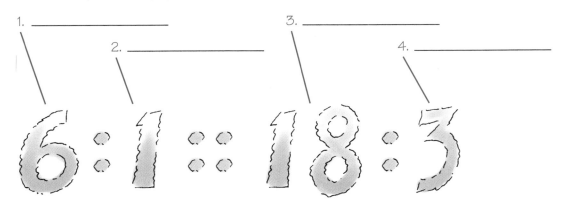

■ Batter's box

Fill in the blanks with the correct information regarding proportions.

A proportion can be written with _____ . The _____ , or end,
                                         1   2

numbers are called the _____ , and the _____ , or middle,
                                   3   4

numbers are called the _____ . In such a proportion, the _____
                                   5   6

of the means _____ the _____ of the extremes.
                        7   8

Options
A. equals
B. inner
C. outer
D. means
E. product
F. ratios
G. product
H. extremes

Jumble gym

Test your dexterity by unscrambling these letters to finish the sentence.

Question: **The product of the means equals the product of the _____ .**

E T M E R E X

Answer: __ __ __ __ __ __ __

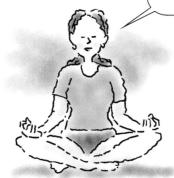

The mind is a terrible thing to waste, so let's use it!

Train your brain

Solve this riddle to find an important fact about solving proportions.

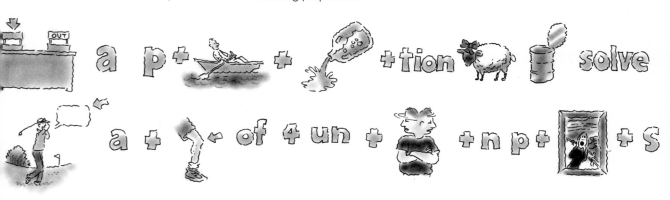

■ Starting lineup

Six steps are needed to solve the equation $X : 20 :: 50 : 10$. Place these steps in their proper order.

$X = 100$	
$1{,}000 \div 10 = X$	
$\dfrac{1{,}000}{10} = \dfrac{10X}{10}$	
$20 \times 50 = X \times 10$	
$100 : 20 :: 50 : 10$	
$1{,}000 = 10X$	

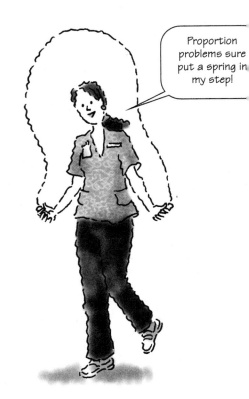

Proportion problems sure put a spring in my step!

■ Hit or miss

We solved for X, now you solve for X. Is the answer we got a direct hit? Label it with a "T" for "True" and an "F" for "False."

$25 : 75 :: X : 33$

$X = 11$

Answer: _____

Finish line

Complete the ratios by filling in the missing part of each problem.

1. $X : 8 :: 9 : 36$

$8 \times 9 = X \times 36$

_____

$72 \div 36 = X$

$X = 2$

$2 : 8 :: 9 : 36$

2. $20 : 100 :: 5 : X$

$100 \times 5 = 20 \times X$

$\dfrac{500}{20} = \dfrac{20X}{20}$

_____

$X = 25$

$20 : 100 :: 5 : 25$

3. $3 : 15 :: X : 50$

$15 \times X = 3 \times 50$

$\dfrac{15X}{15} = \dfrac{150}{15}$

$X = \dfrac{150}{15}$

_____

$3 : 15 :: 10 : 50$

4. $8 : X :: 2 : 16$

_____

$\dfrac{2X}{2} = \dfrac{128}{2}$

$X = \dfrac{128}{2}$

$X = 64$

$8 : 64 :: 2 : 16$

I'm not letting these equations slow me down!

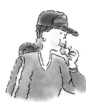

Coaching session
Cross products

In a proportion expressed as fractions, cross products are equal. This means that the numerator on the equation's left side multiplied by the denominator on the equation's right side equals the denominator on the equation's left side multiplied by the numerator on the equation's right side. This illustration represents this principle more simply:

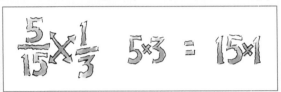

The sample principle applies to proportions expressed as ratios. As shown in this illustration, the product of the **m**eans (numbers in the **m**iddle) equals the products of the **e**xtremes (numbers on the **e**nds).

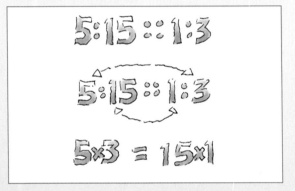

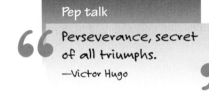

Pep talk

Perseverance, secret of all triumphs.
—Victor Hugo

Multiple reps

Fill in the correct answer.

A physician prescribes 0.125 mg of a drug. The vial the nurse obtains from the pharmacy contains 0.25 mg/ml of solution.

Question: **How many milliliters of the solution should the nurse administer?**

1. 0.5 ml

2. 1 ml

3. 1.5 ml

4. 2 ml

Answer: _____

▪▪
▪ Match point

Part one: Match the steps for solving this problem using ratios to their actual step equivalents.

Question: If a hospital has two registered nurses for every 10 patients, how many registered nurses are needed for 30 patients?

Clues

1. Decide what part of the proportion is X. _____

2. Set up the proportion so that the unit of measure (nurses and patients) in each ratio are in the same position. _____

3. Multiply the means and extremes. _____

4. Set up the equation. _____

5. Solve for X. _____

6. Find X. _____

Options

A. 2 nurses **:** 10 patients **::** X nurses **:** 30 patients

B. $X = \dfrac{60}{10}$

C. 10 patients $\times \dfrac{X}{10 \text{ patients}} = 2$ nurses $\times \dfrac{30 \text{ patients}}{10 \text{ patients}}$

D. $X = 6$ nurses

E. $X =$ number of nurses

F. 10 patients $\times X = 2$ nurses $\times 30$ patients

> Whew! I hope these steps are a little easier than the ones I've been doing!

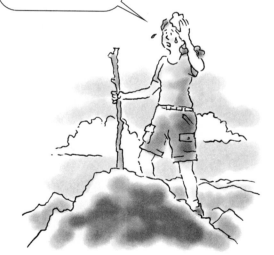

▪▪
▪ Match point

Part two: Now match the steps for solving the same problem using fractions to their actual step equivalents.

Clues

1. Set up the proportion so that the unit of measure is the same in each fraction. _____

2. Rewrite the equation by cross-multiplying the fractions. _____

3. Solve for X. _____

4. Find X. _____

Options

A. 2 nurses $\times \dfrac{30 \text{ patients}}{10 \text{ patients}} = X \times \dfrac{10 \text{ patients}}{10 \text{ patients}}$; $60 \div 10 = X$ nurses

B. 2 nurses $\times 30$ patients $= X$ nurses $\times 10$ patients

C. $X = 6$ nurses

D. $\dfrac{2 \text{ nurses}}{10 \text{ patients}} = \dfrac{X}{30 \text{ patients}}$

Finish line

This equation needs a little pumping up to get to the end. Fill in the missing numbers.

$$\frac{2}{3} = \frac{30}{X}$$

$$2 \times X = 3 \times 30$$

$$2X = \underline{\hspace{1cm}} \quad (1)$$

$$\frac{2X}{2} = \frac{\underline{\hspace{0.8cm}}}{2} \quad (2)$$

$$X = \frac{\underline{\hspace{0.8cm}}}{2} \quad (3)$$

$$X = 45$$

$$\frac{2}{3} = \frac{\underline{\hspace{0.8cm}}}{45} \quad (4)$$

C'mon! Show those blanks who's boss!

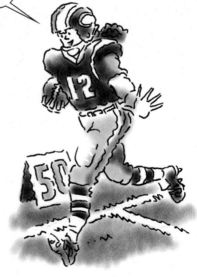

Batter's box

Fill the missing numbers into this equation.

$$\frac{1}{4} = \frac{X}{100}$$

$$1 \times 100 = 4 \times X$$

$$\underline{\hspace{1cm}}_1 = \underline{\hspace{1cm}}_2 \times \underline{\hspace{1cm}}_3$$

$$\frac{100}{4} = \frac{4X}{4}$$

$$\underline{\hspace{1cm}}_4 = \underline{\hspace{1cm}}_5$$

$$\frac{1}{4} = \frac{25}{100}$$

Options

A. X

B. 4

C. X

D. 25

E. 100

■ Batter's box

Fill in the blanks with the correct information regarding dimensional analysis.

Dimensional analysis is also known as _____ analysis or factor

_____ . Dimensional analysis uses the same terms as fractions, specifically
    2

the terms _____ and _____ . When using dimensional analysis,
        3   4

a series of _____ , called factors, are arranged in a fractional equation and
            5

only _____ equation is required to determine each answer.
     6

Options
A. numerator
B. ratios
C. factor
D. denominator
E. labeling
F. one

My dimensions might need some analysis after all this sweating!

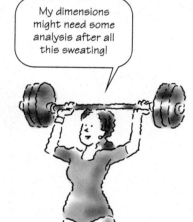

■ Jumble gym

Fill in the missing word by unscrambling these words.

Question: Conversion factors are _____ between two measurement systems or units of measurement.

1. E M P T U E Q I N ◯ _ _ _ _ _ _ ◯◯

2. S M U J P _ ◯ _ _ ◯

3. U A L T V ◯◯ _ ◯ _

4. S Q U P H I E Y _ _ _ _ _ ◯◯ _ ◯

Answer: __ __ __ __ __ __ __ __ __ __ __ __

Match point

Match the unit of measure in Column 1 with its equivalent in Column 2.

Clues

1. 16 oz _____
2. 1 tsp _____
3. 1 kg _____
4. 3' _____
5. 8 oz _____
6. 1 grain _____
7. 1 oz _____
8. 12" _____

Options

A. 5 ml
B. 1 lb
C. 1 yd
D. 2.2 lb
E. 30 ml
F. 1'
G. 60 mg
H. 1 cup

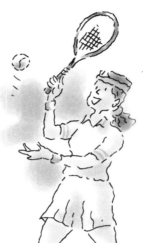

I could really use an ace here.

Strikeout

Strike out the incorrect answers.

Question: If an ounce of prevention is worth a pound of cure, how many milliliters would you need for that cure?

1. 60 ml
2. 90 ml
3. 30 ml
4. There is no cure for this one.

Pep talk

A pessimist sees the difficulty in every opportunity; an optimist sees the opportunity in every difficulty.
—Sir Winston Churchill

■■
■ Hit or miss

Label each statement with a "T" for "True" or an "F" for "False."

_____ 1. 64 oz = 8 cups

_____ 2. 64 oz = 4 lb

_____ 3. 64 oz = 1,920 ml

_____ 4. 64 oz = 2.1 kg

_____ 5. 64 oz = 1.9 L

■■
■ Strikeout

Strike out the incorrect answers.

Question: If your gym bag weighs 20 lb, how many ounces does it weigh?

1. 480 oz

2. 320 oz

3. 340 oz

4. 400 oz

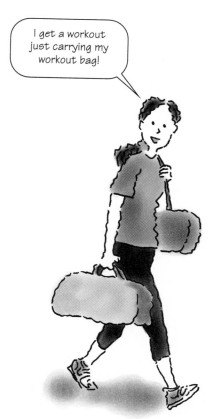

I get a workout just carrying my workout bag!

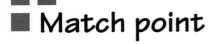

Match point

Match the steps needed to solve this problem with their numerical equivalents.

Question: A doctor prescribes 150 mg of a drug. The pharmacy stocks a solution containing the drug at a concentration of 100 mg/ml. What dose should you give in milliliters?

Clues

Step 1: Given _____

Step 2: Wanted _____

Step 3: Conversion factor _____

Step 4: Set up the equation _____

Step 5: Cancel unwanted units _____

Step 6: Multiply, multiply, and divide _____

Options

A. $\dfrac{150 \cancel{\text{ mg}}}{1} \times \dfrac{1 \text{ ml}}{100 \cancel{\text{ mg}}}$

B. 100 mg = 1 ml

C. $150 \times \dfrac{1 \text{ ml}}{1} \times 100 = \dfrac{150}{100} = 1.5$ ml of the solution

D. 150 mg

E. $\dfrac{150 \text{ mg}}{1} \times \dfrac{1 \text{ ml}}{100 \text{ mg}}$

F. X ml

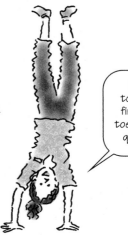

Feel free to use your fingers and toes on these questions!

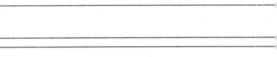

Starting lineup

Put the steps in the order needed to solve this problem.

Question: The doctor prescribes 150 mg of amoxicillin which comes in a suspension of 25 mg/ml. How many teaspoons the suspension should you give?

1 tsp = 5 ml; 25 mg = 1 ml
$\dfrac{1 \text{ tsp}}{5 \cancel{\text{ ml}}} \times \dfrac{1 \cancel{\text{ ml}}}{25 \cancel{\text{ mg}}} \times \dfrac{150 \cancel{\text{ mg}}}{1}$
150 mg
$\dfrac{1 \text{ tsp}}{5 \text{ ml}} \times \dfrac{1 \text{ ml}}{25 \text{ mg}} \times \dfrac{150 \text{ mg}}{1}$
$1 \text{ tsp} \times 1 \times \dfrac{150}{5} \times 25 \times 1 = \dfrac{150 \text{ tsp}}{125} = 1.2$ tsp of the suspension
X tsp

Cross-training

Test your knowledge of math basics with this review.

Across

2. Stands for unknown quantity in an equation
4. End numbers in a ratio
5. Middle numbers in a ratio
7. 1,000 times shorter than a meter

Down

1. To change fractions to decimals
3. Math used to solve for *X*
6. Metric term for weight measurement
8. Metric term for measuring fluid

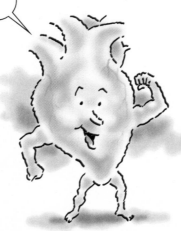

You've finished the first chapter! Are you pumped or what?

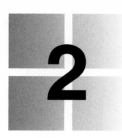

Measurement systems

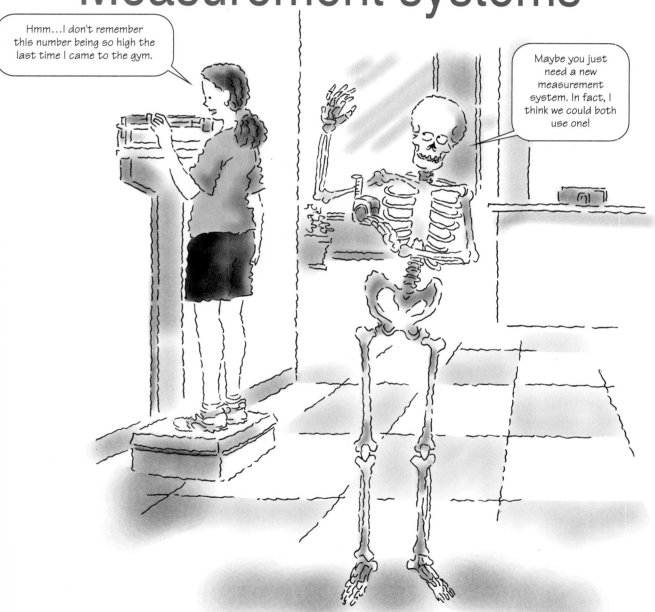

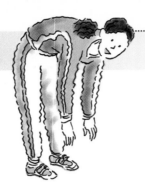

Warm-up

Measurement systems review

Metric basics review

- The metric system is the most widely used system for measuring amounts of drugs.
- It's a decimal system (based on the number 10 and its multiples and subdivisions).
- Three basic units of measurement are used in the metric system
  - meter, basic unit of length
  - liter, basic unit of volume
  - gram, basic unit of weight.
- Multiples and subdivisions of meters, liters, and grams are indicated by using a prefix before the basic units, such as kilo, centi, or milli.

Metric conversions

- To convert a smaller unit to a larger unit:
  - move the decimal point to the left
  - OR divide by the appropriate multiple
  - OR multiply by the appropriate subdivision.

Solving for *X*

- Set up an equation, substituting X for the unknown you're trying to determine.
- Cross-multiply the fractions.
- Divide both sides to isolate X on one side.
- Cancel units that appear in both the numerator and the denominator.
- Do the math!

Metric math

- First, convert all quantities to the same unit.
- Use the common unit that's easiest (unless the problem calls for a specific unit).
- Do the math!

Apothecaries' system

- Measures liquid volume and solid weight
- Minim—basic unit of liquid volume
- Grain—basic unit of solid weight
- 1 drop = 1 minim = 1 grain
- Traditionally uses Roman numerals

Roman numerals

- To convert a Roman numeral to an Arabic numeral:
  - if a smaller Roman numeral precedes a larger Roman numeral, subtract the smaller numeral from the larger numeral
  - if a smaller Roman numeral follows a larger Roman numeral, add the numerals.
- To convert an Arabic numeral to a Roman numeral:
  - break the Arabic numeral into its component parts
  - translate each part into Roman numerals.

Household system

- Uses droppers, teaspoons, and cups to measure liquid medication doses
- Common household conversions:
  3 tsp = 1 tbs
  8 oz = 1 cup
  4 qt = 1 gal

Avoirdupois system

- Pronounced "av-wah-doo-PWAH"
- Solid measures or units of weight, including grains, ounces, and pounds
- Common avoirdupois conversions:
  1 oz = 480 gr
  1 lb = 16 oz = 7,680 gr

Unit conversions

- Insulin is the most common drug measured in units.
- Divide the units required by the amount of drug available in units.

Milliequivalent conversions

- Measures some electrolytes.
- Divide the amount of milliequivalents required by the amount of drug available in milliequivalents.

Commonly used conversions

- Pounds to kilograms: Divide the number of pounds by 2.2.
- Kilograms to pounds: Multiply the number of kilograms by 2.2.
- Inches to centimeters: Multiply the number of inches by 2.54.
- Centimeters to inches: Divide the number of centimeters by 2.54.

■ Cross-training

Test your knowledge of the metric system with this review.

Across

3. The metric system simplifies the calculation of this kind of dose.
5. Type of system used worldwide for measurement
7. The metric system eliminates this type of fraction.

Down

1. The basic metric unit of length
2. The basic metric unit of volume
3. Metric measurements use this type of system.
4. The basic metric unit of weight
6. The metric system simplifies the calculation of large and small _____ .

I wish I could use metrics to simplify my workout routine!

Gear up!

Pick out which tools you'll need to measure in metrics.

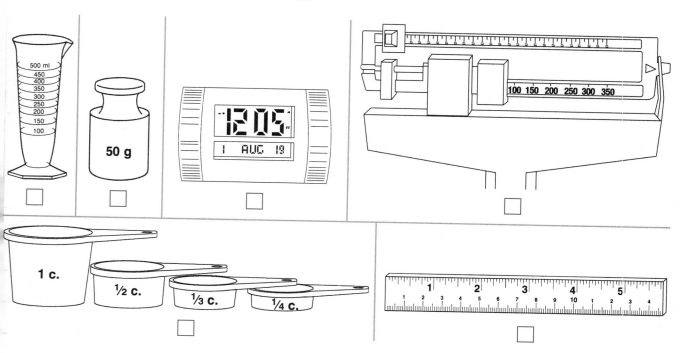

Match point

Match the metric system prefix with its corresponding abbreviation.

Clues

1. kilo _____
2. hecto _____
3. deka _____
4. deci _____
5. centi _____
6. milli _____
7. micro _____
8. nano _____
9. pico _____

Options

A. dk
B. c
C. mc
D. p
E. k
F. d
G. h
H. m
I. n

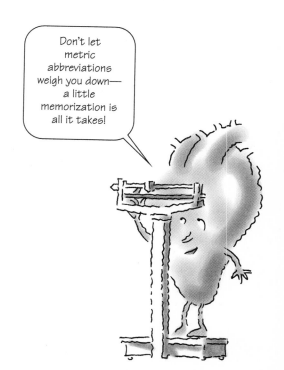

Don't let metric abbreviations weigh you down—a little memorization is all it takes!

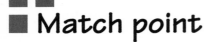

Match point

Match the abbreviation with its corresponding multiple or subdivision.

Clues

1. k _____
2. h _____
3. dk _____
4. d _____
5. c _____
6. m _____
7. mc _____
8. n _____
9. p _____

Options

A. 0.000000000001 ($\frac{1}{1,000,000,000,000}$)
B. 100
C. 0.01 ($\frac{1}{100}$)
D. 1,000
E. 0.001 ($\frac{1}{1,000}$)
F. 0.000000001 ($\frac{1}{1,000,000,000}$)
G. 0.1 ($\frac{1}{10}$)
H. 0.000001 ($\frac{1}{1,000,000}$)
I. 10

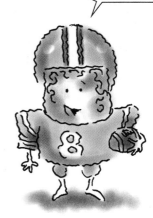

This game is making you go the whole nine yards! By the way, that's 8.2296 meters.

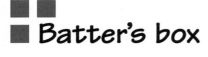

Batter's box

Fill in the correct measuring tool from the options listed for each of these items. Note that you'll have to repeat some options.

Clues

1. Water _____
2. Cocoa powder _____
3. Sears Tower _____
4. Petroleum jelly _____
5. Wine _____
6. Football field _____
7. Air _____
8. Sand _____

Options

A. Metric weights
B. Metric graduate
C. Metric ruler

Train your brain

Solve this riddle to find an important fact about units of volume.

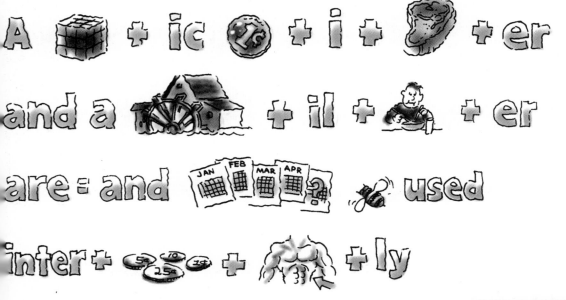

Hit or miss

Label each statement with a "T" for "True" or an "F" for "False."

___ 1. To convert a smaller unit to a larger unit, move the decimal point to the right.

___ 2. To convert a larger unit to a smaller unit, multiply by the appropriate multiple or divide by the appropriate subdivision.

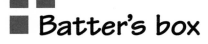

Batter's box

Fill in the blanks with the correct information regarding metric conversions.

Liquids	Solids
1 ml = _____ (1)	_____ (6) = 1 mg
1,000 ml = 1 L	1,000 mg = 1 g
_____ (2) = 1 L	100 cg = _____ (7)
1 dl = _____ (3)	10 dg = 1 g
10 L = 1 dkl	10 g = _____ (8)
100 L = _____ (4)	100 g = _____ (9)
_____ (5) = 1 kl	_____ (10) = 1 kg

Options

A. 1 hl

B. 1 g

C. 100 cl

D. 1,000 g

E. 1,000 mcg

F. 1 dkg

G. 1 cm³ (or cc)

H. 1 hg

I. 1,000 L

J. 1 L

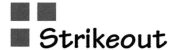

Strikeout

Strike out the incorrect answers.

Question: The finish line is 3 km away. How many meters is that?

1. 30 m

2. 300 m

3. 3,000 m

4. 30,000 m

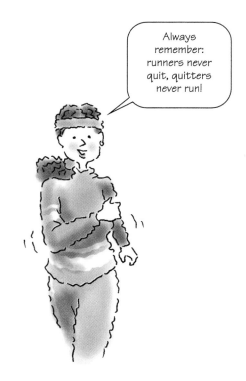

Always remember: runners never quit, quitters never run!

Hit or miss

Label each statement with a "T" for "True" and an "F" for "False."

_____ 1. Time out for a chocolate break! Your chocolate reward weighs 30,000 mg. But don't worry; that works out to a mere 300 g.

_____ 2. A patient received 5 grams of a drug. In other words, he received 5,000 mg.

> **Pep talk**
>
> " If a man does his best, what else is there?
> —General George S. Patton "

Multiple reps

Fill in the correct answer.

Question: You're whipping up some smoothies. The recipe calls for 2 kg of bananas, 3,000 mg of strawberries, and 10 g of kiwi. How many total grams of fruit do you need?

A. 2,013

B. 2,310

C. 2,040

D. 2,301

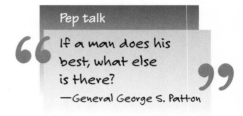

I'll need lots of fruit to replace these lost calories. Bring on the kilos!

Answer: _____

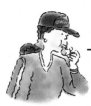

Coaching session
For fraction phobes

If working with fractions puts you in a sweat, here's another way to solve for X in problems. Let's say an infant weighs 6.5 kg and you need to find out how much he weighs in grams. You can set this up as a ratio and proportion instead of a fraction:

$$1,000 \text{ g} : 1 \text{ kg} :: X : 6.5 \text{ kg}$$

- Multiply the means and extremes:

$$X \times 1 \text{ kg} = 1,000 \text{ g} \times 6.5 \text{ kg}$$

- Divide both sides of the equation by 1 kg to isolate X.
- Cancel units that appear in both the numerator and denominator.

$$X = 6,500 \text{ g}$$

The infant weighs 6,500 g.

Now, remember to hit 'em with your cross here. I mean cross-multiplication, of course.

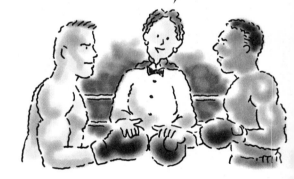

Starting lineup

Put the steps in the order needed to solve this problem.

Your patient needs 300,000 units by I.M. injection. The vial of penicillin that's available contains 1,000,000 units/ml. How much of the drug should you draw up?

$X \times 1,000,000 \text{ units} = 1 \text{ ml} \times 300,000 \text{ units}$	
$X = 0.3 \text{ ml}$	
$X \times \dfrac{1,000,000 \text{ units}}{1,000,000 \text{ units}} = 1 \text{ ml} \times \dfrac{300,000 \text{ units}}{1,000,000 \text{ units}}$	
$\dfrac{X}{300,000 \text{ units}} = \dfrac{1 \text{ ml}}{1,000,000 \text{ units}}$	

Finish line

Fill in the missing parts of the calculation that solves this problem.

Your patient needs 20 mEq of sodium bicarbonate. The vial from the pharmacy contains 50 mEq in 50 ml. How many milliliters of the solution should you administer?

$$\frac{X}{20 \text{ mEq}} = \frac{}{50 \text{ mEq}} \quad (1)$$

$$X \times 50 \text{ mEq} = 50 \text{ ml} \times \underline{\hspace{1cm}} \quad (2)$$

$$X \times \frac{\cancel{50 \text{ mEq}}}{\cancel{50 \text{ mEq}}} = 50 \text{ ml} \times \frac{20 \cancel{\text{ mEq}}}{50 \cancel{\text{ mEq}}}$$

$$X = \underline{\hspace{1cm}} \quad (3)$$

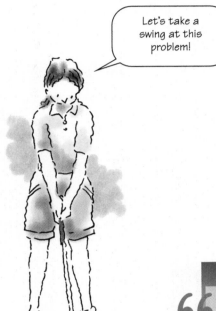

Let's take a swing at this problem!

Jumble gym

Unscramble each word to discover terms related to the unit system. Then use the circled letters to answer the question below.

Question: **Which drug is most commonly measured in units?**

1. S I T N U _ ◯ ◯ _ _

2. N O V I C E S N O R _ _ _ _ _ _ _ ◯ _ _ ◯

3. A I N A N E R L I N T T O   I T S U N

◯ _ _ _ _ _ _ _ _ _ _ _ ◯ ◯ _ _ _ _

Answer: _ _ _ _ _ _ _ _

■■ ■ Hit or miss

Is the following statement true or false? Label it with a "T" for "True" or an "F" for "False."

It's the physician's responsibility to provide information about the number of metric units required to provide the prescribed number of milliequivalents.

Answer: _____

■■ ■ Finish line

Does your conversion knowledge measure up? Fill in the missing values to find out.

Liquids	Household	Apothecaries'	Metric
	1 drop (gtt)	1 minim (m)	___1___ milliliter (ml)
	15 to 16 gtt	15 to 16 m	___2___ ml
	___3___ teaspoon (tsp)	1 fluidram	5 ml
	1 tablespoon (tbs)	___4___ fluid ounce (oz)	15 ml
	___5___ tbs	1 fluid oz	30 ml
	1 cup	___6___ fluid oz	240 ml
	1 pint (pt)	16 fluid oz	___7___ ml
	1 quart (qt)	___8___ fluid oz	960 ml
	1 gallon (gal)	128 fluid oz	___9___ ml

Solids	Avoirdupois	Apothecaries'	Metric
	1 grain (gr)	1 gr	___10___ (g)
	1 gr	1 gr	___11___ milligrams (mg)
	15.4 gr	___12___ gr	1 g
	1 oz	___13___ gr	28.35 g
	___14___ pound (lb)	1.33 lb	454 g
	2.2 lb	___15___ lb	1 kilogram (kg)

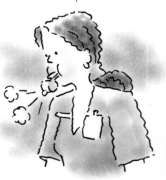

Game over! Take a minute to rest up before you hit chapter 3.

3

Recording drug administration

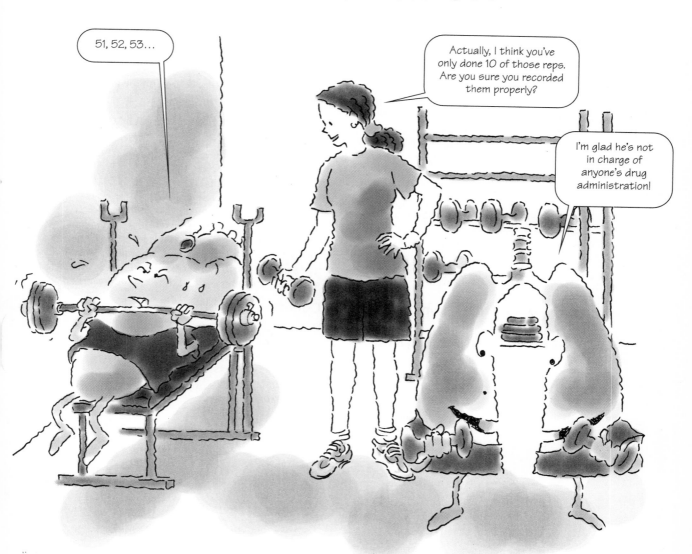

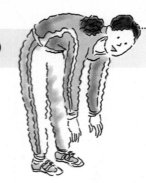

Recording drug administration review

Reading and transcribing drug orders

Make sure the drug order includes all of the following information:
- drug name
- dose
- administration route
- time and frequency of administration.

Using military time

- To write single-digit times from 1:00 a.m. to 9:59 a.m., put a zero before the time and remove the colon.
- To write double-digit times from 10:00 a.m. to 12:59 p.m., just remove the colon.
- To write times from 1:00 p.m. to 12 a.m. (midnight), add 1200 to the hour and remove the colon.
- To write times from 12:01 a.m. to 12:59 a.m., remove the 12 and colon and replace with 00.
- Minutes after the hour remain the same.

Administering drugs

- Give drug within 30 minutes of the specified time.
- Record the actual administration time.
- If the drug is discontinued, make sure the practitioner writes a new order.
- With each order, ensure that the appropriate drug is being administered.

Drug administration record systems

- Medical administration record
  - Uses a form to record medication administration
  - Widely used
- Computer charting
  - Medication administration information entered into a computer
  - Automatic, computer-generated list of scheduled medications and their administration times
  - Used increasingly more over other systems

Documenting drug administration

- Write legibly in blue or black ink.
- Record allergy information if it isn't already documented.
- Transcribe from the practitioner's order complete information about each drug (dates and drug names, dosages, strengths, dosage forms, administration routes, and administration times).
- If parenteral, record the injection site.
- Immediately document the times of all administrations.
- If unscheduled, record the exact time the drug was given.
- If given late or not at all, document the reason.
- Always sign any documentation on the administration record.

Recording controlled-substance administration

- Include date and time dose is removed from locked storage area.
- Include amount of drug remaining in locked storage area.
- Record the patient's full name.
- Document the practitioner's full name.
- Enter the drug dose given.
- Include your full signature (if a form is used; the nurse's password serves as a signature if a computer is used).
- If any part of the drug was discarded, obtain the signature of another nurse who verified the amount discarded.

Common drug errors

- Dosage calculation errors
- Drug name errors
- Patient name errors
- Missed allergy alerts
- Compound errors
- Route errors
- Misinterpreted orders
- Preparation errors
- Stress-related errors

Avoiding transcription errors

- Transcribe orders in a quiet area.
- Carefully check your work before signing.
- Follow your facility's policy for reviewing orders.

Refusing to carry out an order

- Notify your supervisor.
- Notify the prescribing practitioner.
- Document according to your facility's policy.

The five "rights" of drug administration

- Right drug
- Right dose
- Right route
- Right time
- Right patient

In cases of error

- Notify the practitioner.
- Consult the pharmacist.
- Assess the patient throughout.
- Follow your facility's drug error documentation policy.

■ Match point

Match the drug order information with its correct description.

Clues

1. P.O., I.M., I.V., P.R., or S.L. _____
2. Times per day or hours between doses _____
3. Dosage form _____
4. Practitioner's registration number _____
5. Name of drug _____
6. Drug order sheet _____

Options

A. Written in metric, apothecaries', or household measuremen
B. Necessary for controlled drugs, if applicable
C. When to administer drug
D. Abbreviation for the route of administration
E. Usually stamped with patient's admission data plate
F. Can be generic or trade

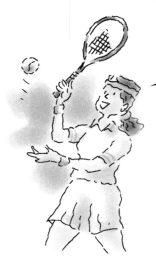

Master drug order data to be at the top of your game!

■ Strikeout

Strike out the clocks that don't have the correct time listed.

1.
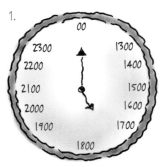
It's 6 a.m.

2.
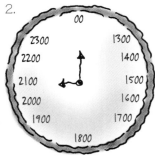
It's 9 p.m.

3.

It's 0200 hours.

4.

It's 1300 hours.

■■ ■ Hit or miss

Label each statement with a "T" for "True" or an "F" for "False."

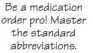

Be a medication order pro! Master the standard abbreviations.

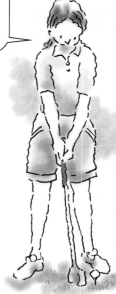

_____ 1. You should use "cc" to abbreviate "cubic centimeter."

_____ 2. "Fluid ounce" is abbreviated as "fl oz."

_____ 3. "Liter" is abbreviated as "l."

_____ 4. "Capsule" is abbreviated as "cap."

_____ 5. "DS" is the abbreviation for "double solution."

_____ 6. "Long-acting" is abbreviated as "LA."

_____ 7. "A.D." is the abbreviation for "right ear," and "A.U." is the abbreviation for "each ear."

_____ 8. "P.R." means "rectally," and "P.V." means "vaginally."

_____ 9. "Before meals" is abbreviated as "a.c."

_____ 10. The abbreviation "q4H" stands for "every four hours."

■■ ■ Finish line

Take these crunched versions of practitioners' drug orders and stretch them out into their full instruction form.

Brenda Pillola, M.D.
123 Main Street
Wellville, PA 00100
(800) 555-4321

℞

Glucophage 500 mg P.O. b.i.d. a.c.

Brenda Pillola, MD

1. _____

_____

Brenda Pillola, M.D.
123 Main Street
Wellville, PA 00100
(800) 555-4321

℞

Begin clopidogrel 75 mg P.O. daily.

Brenda Pillola, MD

2. _____

_____

Brenda Pillola, M.D.
123 Main Street
Wellville, PA 00100
(800) 555-4321

℞

Increase Demerol to 25 mg I.V. q4h.

Brenda Pillola, MD

3. _____

_____

Brenda Pillola, M.D.
123 Main Street
Wellville, PA 00100
(800) 555-4321

℞

Lisinopril 10 mg P.O. q8h; hold for SBP less than 90.

Brenda Pillola, MD

4. _____

_____

Brenda Pillola, M.D.
123 Main Street
Wellville, PA 00100
(800) 555-4321

℞

Discontinue famotidine I.V.

Brenda Pillola, MD

5. _____

_____

Brenda Pillola, M.D.
123 Main Street
Wellville, PA 00100
(800) 555-4321

℞

Temazepam 12.5-25 mg P.O. at bedtime p.r.n. sleeplessness.

Brenda Pillola, MD

6. _____

_____

Jumble gym

Unscramble each word to discover the information you need to transcribe from the practitioner's order to the medication administration record (MAR). Then use the circled letters to answer the question below.

Question: **What do you need to do on the MAR to indicate that you've carried out the practitioner's order?**

1. T E A D ◯ _ _ _

2. M A N E _ _ ◯ _

3. T T S E G H N R _ ◯ _ _ _ _ _ _

4. R O M F _ ◯ _ _

5. U O R E T _ _ ◯ _ _

6. T I E S _ _ _ ◯

7. L E S U H C E D _ ◯ _ _ _ _ _ _

8. R E I A N T U G S _ _ _ ◯ _ _ _ _ _

Answer: _ _ _ _ _ _ _ _

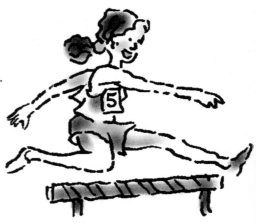

Now that you've learned how to document on the MAR, you're really going strong!

Strikeout

Strike out the incorrect statements.

1. If a drug order seems questionable, only ask the pharmacist to check it.

2. You should always use the five "rights" before giving a drug.

3. You should check and recheck all your drug calculations.

4. It's ok to administer a drug from a vial without a label.

5. You should never use open or unmarked I.V. solution bags.

Batter's box

Fill in the blanks with the correct information regarding medication administration records.

. The date the prescription was _____ .

. The date drug administration should _____ .

. The date the drug should be _____ .

. The drug's full _____ name.

. Don't use _____ for drug names.

. Don't use _____ symbols for drug names.

. When recording drug strength, be sure to write the _____ amount of the drug to be administered.

Options

A. actual

B. begin

C. written

D. discontinued

E. generic

F. chemical

G. abbreviations

Hit or miss

Label each statement with a "T" for "True" or an "F" for "False."

____ 1. Some facilities have computerized drug dispensing systems on every unit.

____ 2. One type of computerized drug dispensing system is called *Pyxis*.

____ 3. Computerized drug dispensing systems dispense regular medications, but not controlled substances.

____ 4. Your username only serves as your signature.

____ 5. Your username and password serve as your signature.

____ 6. You don't need another nurse to witness any part of a controlled substance you discard.

____ 7. The system will usually display a prompt screen for another nurse to enter her username and password if you discard a controlled substance.

Computerized drug dispensing systems make your job easier. You'll be cycling around quicker than ever!

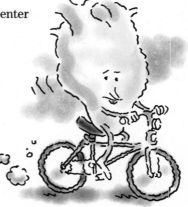

Cross-training

Here's an exercise to help expand your knowledge of drug administration.

Across

4. You should _____ the actual administration time.

6. With each order, ensure that the _____ drug is being administered.

7. All drug orders must follow a specific _____ .

Down

1. Record on the MAR the date the drug is started and _____ .

2. The first item in standard sequence is the drug _____ .

3. Give the drug within _____ minutes of the specified time.

5. Drugs can be ordered by _____ the order to the pharmacy.

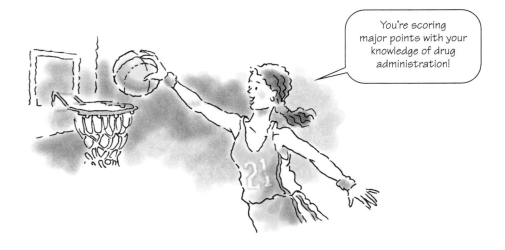

You're scoring major points with your knowledge of drug administration!

Finish line

Refer to this chart to fill in the answers to the following questions about medication records.

Initial	Signature	Initial	Signature
JH	John Haney, RN	CK	Colleen Kelly, RN
CJ	Chris Johnson, RN	LW	Lori Whittaker, RN

MARY JANE TURNER
42 Penn St
Well, PA 82547
Unit: 2 North 212 B

Allergies
Aspirin

R = Refused   O = Omitted   F = Fasting

Date ordered	Stop date	Medication / Dose / Route / Frequency	R.N. initial	Time	9/15	9/16	9/17	9/18	9/19	9/20	
9/15/08	9/20/08	digoxin 0.125 mg P.O.	JH	0900	JH	JH					
9/15/08	9/20/08	furosemide 40 mg P.O. b.i.d.		0900	JH	JH					
			JH	2100	CK	CK					
9/15/08	9/20/08	glyburide 2.5 mg P.O. qa.m.	JH	0800	JH	JH					
9/15/08	9/20/08	famotidine 20 mg I.V. q 12 h		0900	/	JH					
			JH	2100	JH	LW					
9/16/08	9/19/08	heparin sodium 5000 units subQ q 12 h		0600	/	/					
			JH	1800	/	CK					

Routine medications

Diagnosis and Surgery: Fem pop bypass
Age: 60
Sex: F
Physician: A. R. Tree
Room: 212 B
Name: Mary Jane Turner

FREEDOM HOSPITAL

1. Which medications should be administered at 9 a.m.? _____

2. Which medication should be administered at 6 a.m.? _____

3. According to the medication record, can the nurse administer glyburide on 9/21? _____

4. By which route should the nurse administer digoxin? _____

5. Is this patient allergic to any medications? _____

6. Which medication should be administered at 6 p.m.? _____

7. The patient was supposed to receive furosemide 40 mg P.O. at 9 p.m. on 9/16. However, this dose was omitted. Is the documentation on the MAR adequate? _____

8. After administering famotidine as prescribed, the nurses initialed the appropriate blocks. Is their documentation complete? _____

9. Because surgery is schedule at 10 a.m. on 9/17, the patient must remain NPO and miss the 8 a.m. and 9 a.m. doses of the prescribed oral medications on that day. How should the nurse document this on the MAR? _____

■ Batter's box

Fill in the blanks with the correct information regarding common types of drug errors and their causes.

Part 1: Types of errors

1. Giving the wrong _____ , _____ , or _____ .
2. Missing a dose or _____ to give an ordered drug.
3. Giving the drug at the wrong _____ .
4. Administering a drug to which the patient is _____ .
5. Infusing the drug too _____ .
6. Giving the drug to the _____ patient.
7. Administering the drug by the wrong _____ .

Options

A. failing
B. diluent
C. route
D. drug
E. dose
F. wrong
G. rapidly
H. time
I. allergic

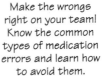

Make the wrongs right on your team! Know the common types of medication errors and learn how to avoid them.

Part 2: Causes

1. Use of _____ stock medications.
2. Failure to follow _____ policies and procedures.
3. Incorrect _____ or administration techniques.
4. Use of I.V. solutions that aren't _____ .
5. Failure to verify drug and dosage _____ .
6. Following _____ , not written, orders.
7. Inadequate _____ .
8. Use of acronyms or erroneous _____ .

Options

A. premixed
B. facility
C. abbreviations
D. floor
E. staffing
F. verbal
G. instructions
H. preparation

Match point

Match the drug names in the first column that sound or look like the drug names in the second column.

Clues

1. Zantac _____
2. Rifadin _____
3. rimantadine _____
4. Celexa _____
5. norepinephrine _____
6. Thorazine _____
7. amiloride _____
8. Zyprexa _____
9. vincristine _____
10. Inderal _____
11. desipramine _____
12. Phenobarbital _____
13. sulfasalazine _____
14. nicardipine _____
15. morphine _____

Options

A. amantadine
B. amiodarone
C. Celebrex
D. Compazine
E. epinephrine
F. hydromorphone
G. imipramine
H. Imuran
I. nifedipine
J. pentobarbital
K. Ritalin
L. sulfisoxazole
M. vinblastine
N. Xanax
O. Zyrtec

Pep talk

"It is no good to try to stop knowledge from going forward. Ignorance is never better than knowledge."

—Enrico Fermi

Double checking the drug names that seem to "match" will help you prevent drug errors.

■■ ■ Batter's box

Fill in the blanks with the correct information regarding drug errors.

Both morphine and hydromorphone are available in _____ prefilled
₁

syringes and both cause _____ depression. However, _____
₂ ₃

has a greater effect on a patient's respiratory status. If you administer morphine when the

prescriber ordered _____ , the patient could develop respiratory depression
₄

or even _____ .
₅

Options
A. hydromorphone
B. arrest
C. 4 mg
D. respiratory
E. morphine

> With a steady stream of drug names that look and sound alike, getting the right drug requires a careful balancing act.

■■ ■ Hit or miss

Is the following statement true or false? Label it with a "T" for "True" or an "F" for "False."

Question: When double-checking that drug orders are going to the right patient, you should always check the patient's name against his chart and identification bracelet.

Answer: _____

■ Finish line

Refer to this chart to fill in the answers to the following questions about medication records.

Initial	Signature	Initial	Signature
SA	Sally Adamson, RN		
JJ	Jean Johnson, RN		

JOSEPH JACKSON
33 Short Street
Hope, NJ 22124
Unit: 4 South 432 A

Allergies
_____ Aspirin _____

R = Refused   O = Omitted   F = Fasting

Date ordered	Stop date	Medication / Dose / Route / Frequency	R.N. initial	Time	2/14	2/15	2/16	2/17	2/18	2/19
2/14/08	2/19/08	carbidopa/levidopa 25/250 P.O. b.i.d.	SA	0900 2100	X					
2/14/08	2/19/08	benztropine 1.0 mg P.O. t.i.d.	SA	1000 1400 1800	X					
2/14/08	2/16/08	diphenhydramine 25 mg P.O. at bedtime	SA	2200						

Routine medications

Diagnosis and Surgery: Pneumonia
Age: 72
Sex: M
Physician: Dr. Novak
Room: 432A
Name: Joseph Jackson

FREEDOM HOSPITAL

1. Which medications should be administered at 9 a.m.? _____

2. Which medication should be administered at 6 p.m.? _____

3. According to the medication record, can the nurse administer diphenhydramine on 2/18? _____

4. By which route should the nurse administer benztropine? _____

5. Is this patient allergic to any medications? _____

6. Because surgery is scheduled at 11:00 a.m. on 2/15, the patient must remain NPO and miss the 9 a.m. and 10 a.m. doses of the prescribed oral medications on that day. How should the nurse document this on the MAR? _____
_____

■ Jumble gym

Fill in the blanks to describe ways of preventing drug errors through patient teaching.

1. Teach the patient to offer his _____ bracelet for inspection.

    A C O I F E D I I N N T I T

2. Teach the patient to state his _____ and last name.

    F T S R I

3. The patient should state his name when _____ enters his room.

    N A Y E O N

4. Urge the patient to tell a nurse when his _____ is removed.

    L A C B E R E T

5. _____ a removed bracelet immediately.

    P A C R E E L

> Teaching patients about identification will get you off to a good start in preventing drug errors.

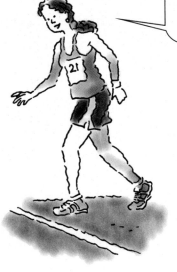

■ Strikeout

Strike out the elements that patients should *not* be taught about in regard to their medications.

1. What medications look like

2. How medications are listed on the medication administration record

3. What times medications should be taken

4. When patients should discontinue medications before checking with a practitioner

5. How medications are given

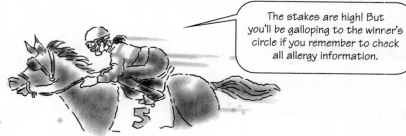

The stakes are high! But you'll be galloping to the winner's circle if you remember to check all allergy information.

Starting lineup

When checking for patient allergies, you need to look for allergy information in certain areas, and in a certain order. Place these steps in their preferred order.

Ask the patient directly about allergies, even if he's in distress.
Verify patient's full name.
Look for allergy medication on the front of the chart or on the medication record.
Double check the allergy information against the chart.
Check to see if he's wearing allergy identification.

Finish line

Take these crunched versions of practitioners' drug orders and stretch them out into their full instruction form.

1. Compazine 5 mg I.M. q 6 h p.r.n for N/V

_____

_____

2. digoxin 0.25 mg P.O. daily, hold for apical pulse less than 60

_____

_____

3. lidocaine 50 mg I.V. bolus at 25 mg/min STAT and q 8–10 min × 1 p.r.n.

_____

_____

4. nifedipine 20 mg SL q 8 h

_____

_____

5. hydroxyzine 25 mg I.M. q 4 h p.r.n. anxiety

_____

_____

Batter's box

Fill in the blanks with the correct information regarding distressing situations.

Any time you're in a tense situation with a patient who needs or wants medication fast,

resist the temptation to _____ first and _____ later. Skipping
                                        1   2

this crucial _____ can lead to a medication _____ .
                      3   4

Options

A. verify

B. error

C. act

D. step

Can I claim an
allergy to
abdominal
exercise?

Hit or miss

Label each statement with a "T" for "True" or an "F" for "False."

_____ 1. Certain medications should never be given to a patient allergic to soy, peanuts, or sulfa compounds.

_____ 2. If a patient has a peanut or soy allergy, you'll need to give him the nasal spray or inhalation solution form of ipratropium (Atrovent).

_____ 3. Patients allergic to sulfa drugs can still receive sulfonylurea hypoglycemic agents.

Starting lineup

Put these steps in the order in which they must proceed for a drug to be given correctly and to avoid compound errors.

The nurse must evaluate whether the medication is appropriate for the patient, then administer it correctly according to facility guidelines.

The practitioner must choose the right medication for the patient, then write the order correctly and legibly.

The pharmacist must interpret the order, determine whether it's complete, and prepare the drug using precise measurements.

> Work together to avoid all types of errors. How about a team cheer?

Jumble gym

Unscramble the terms related to compound errors to answer the question below.

Question: Which important member of the health care team can clarify the number of times a drug can be given in a day?

1. D O C O M P U N ◯ _ _ ◯ _ _ _ _

2. A I C E D I N T O M ◯ _ _ ◯ _ ◯ _ _ _ _

3. R E R R O _ _ ◯ _ _

4. M E T A ◯ _ ◯ _

5. L O B D U E - C E K H C _ _ _ _ _ _ _ _ - _ ◯ _ _ _

6. S R D G U _ _ _ _ ◯

Answer: _ _ _ _ _ _ _ _ _ _

Strikeout

Strike out the statement that *doesn't* describe the nurse's role in preventing drug errors.

1. Preparing the drug using precise measurements
2. Clarifying a practitioner's order that doesn't seem clear or correct
3. Correctly handling and storing multi-dose vials obtained from the pharmacist
4. Administering only those drugs you've personally prepared
5. Choosing the right medication for the patient

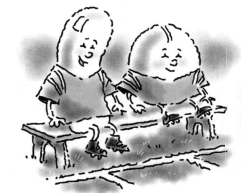

We can't do it alone. We're all in this together!

Hit or miss

Is this statement true or false? Label it with a "T" for "True" or an "F" for "False."

Question: A nurse working in the neonatal intensive care unit prepares a dose of aminophylline to administer to an infant. She clarifies the order with the practitioner before administering it. In a situation like this, the nurse's actions are considered the best practice.

Answer: _____

Batter's box

Fill in the blanks with the correct information regarding making route errors.

Prepare all liquid oral medications in a _____ 1 that has a tip small enough to fit into an _____ 2 tube but too large to fit into a _____ 3 line. Never increase the _____ 4 rate to clear _____ 5 from a line. Instead, remove the _____ 6 from the pump, disconnect it from the _____ 7 , and use the _____ 8 clamp to establish gravity flow of the I.V. fluid to purge air from the line.

> **Options**
> A. flow-control
> B. syringe
> C. abdominal
> D. drip
> E. tubing
> F. bubbles
> G. patient
> H. central

Match point

Match the potential problem in Column 1 with an option from the list of "Do not use" abbreviations in Column 2.

Clues

1. Mistaken as I.V. or 10 _____
2. Confused for one another _____
3. Mistaken for other meaning _____
4. Mistaken for units when poorly written _____
5. Mistaken as "discontinue" _____
6. Mistaken as 0, 4, or cc _____

Options

A. U
B. IU
C. MS, MSO_4, $MgSO_4$
D. h.s.
E. cc
F. D/C

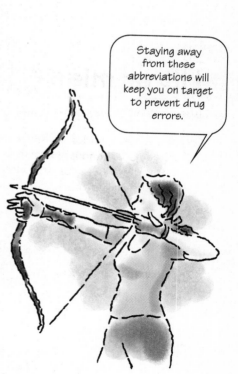

Staying away from these abbreviations will keep you on target to prevent drug errors.

■■ ■ Hit or miss

Label each statement with a "T" for "True" or an "F" for "False."

_____ 1. Even during emergencies, such as a patient resuscitation, verbal orders to administer a drug aren't permitted.

_____ 2. If the order is verbal, you should always repeat it back to the practitioner.

_____ 3. It isn't necessary to document verbal orders on the patient's chart.

_____ 4. You should make sure that the practitioner reviews and signs all orders as necessary.

_____ 5. Some facilities no longer permit verbal orders and telephone orders due to the prevalence of computers at nurse's stations.

■■ ■ Batter's box

Fill in blanks with the correct information regarding preferred terms in The Joint Commission's "Do-not-use" list.

1. Writing _____ is preferred to writing IU.

2. Writing _____ is preferred to writing Q.D.

3. Writing _____ is preferred to writing t.i.w.

4. Writing _____ is preferred to writing D/C.

5. Writing _____ for milliliters is preferred to writing cc for cubic centimeters.

> Options
> A. three times weekly
> B. ml
> C. International Unit
> D. discharge
> E. daily

> Don't turn yourself upside down by using the wrong abbreviations.

■■
■ Batter's box

Fill in the blanks with the correct information regarding preparation errors.

If you notice that a familiar drug has an _____ appearance, you should question
1

the _____ . If he says it's due to a change in _____ , you should
2   3

ask him to double-check whether or not he's received _____ of that change.
4

Make sure to document in the patient's _____ the appearance
5

_____ , your _____ , and the pharmacist's _____ .
6   7   8

Options
A. discrepancy
B. manufacturer
C. record
D. response
E. unfamiliar
F. actions
G. pharmacist
H. verification

> Let's meditate on
> reducing your risk of
> making errors.

■■
■ Jumble gym

Unscramble each word to discover how you should avoid making stress-related drug errors. Then use the circled letters
to answer the question below.

Question: What is one major cause of drug-related errors?

1. L E I S I B Y P N I T O R S _ _ ◯ _ _ _ ◯ _ _ _ _ _ _ _

2. R E R S O R _ _ _ _ _ ◯

3. Z I N E M M I I _ _ _ _ _ _ _ ◯

4. D U G R _ ◯ _ _

5. S I A M A O R N T I I T N D _ _ _ _ _ _ _ _ ◯ _ _ _ _ _ _

Answer: _ _ _ _ _ _ _

■■ Batter's box

Fill in the blanks with the correct information regarding transcription errors.

Transcribe all orders from the practitioner's order sheet to the administration record in a

_____ area, where you can concentrate without interruption. Before

1

_____ the order sheet and _____ the administration record,

2   3

carefully _____ both forms to make sure that you've copied the

4

_____ accurately. Follow your facility's _____ for reviewing

5   6

orders.

Options
A. check
B. signing
C. quiet
D. policy
E. initialing
F. orders

> Maintain your momentum by following guidelines.

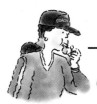

Coaching session
Conquering confusion

Before giving any drug, it's important to review these areas of drug order information:

■ the five rights—make sure that you're giving the right drug, at the right dose, by the right route, at the right time, and to the right patient

■ the math—check your calculations at least twice

■ the label—examine all drug labels closely

■ the name—verify that the drug about to be administered hasn't been confused with one of a similar-sounding or similar-looking name.

Strikeout

Strike out the reasons for which you *can't* legally refuse to administer a drug order.

1. You think that the prescribed dosage is too high.

2. Administering the drug is against your religious or ethical beliefs.

3. You think the patient's physical condition contraindicates use of the drug.

4. You think that the prescribed dosage is too low.

5. You think that the patient would be better helped by a different drug instead.

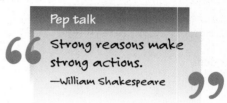

Pep talk

Strong reasons make strong actions.
—William Shakespeare

Starting lineup

Order the steps you should take after making a drug order error.

Follow your facility's policy for documenting drug errors.	
Consult the pharmacist.	
Consider reporting the error to the United States Pharmacopeia.	
Notify the practitioner.	

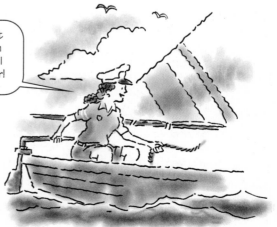

Learning more about drug administration really helped you sail through this chapter!

4

Oral, topical, and rectal drugs

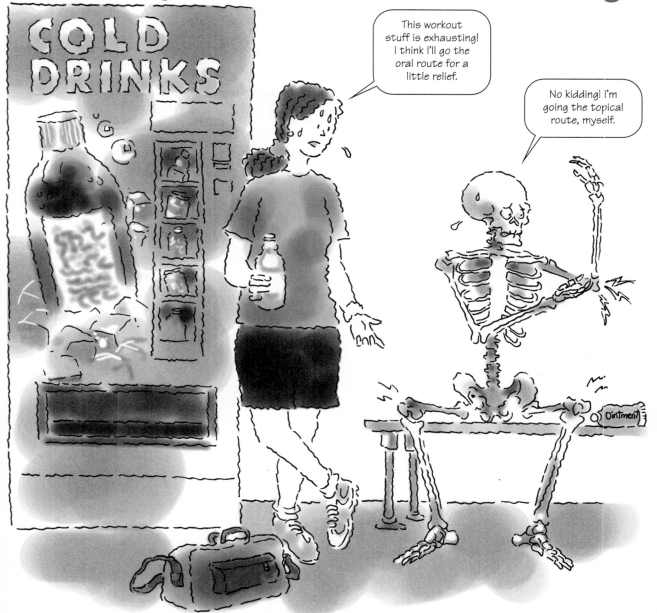

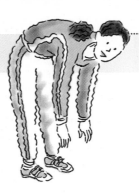

■■ ■ Warm-up

Oral, topical, and rectal drugs review

Reading oral drug labels

■ First, check the drug's generic name and trade name. Remember that combination drugs are usually ordered using the trade name.
■ Then check the dose strength.
■ Lastly, check the expiration date.

Safe oral drug administration

■ Check the "five rights" of medication administration.
■ Check drug names.
■ Check the dosage, route, and medication administration record.
■ Check orders and labels three times.

Dosage calculation key

■ Use correct units of measure.
■ Double-check units of measure and decimal places.
■ Check answers that seem wrong.
■ Use a calculator.

Liquid dosages

■ Read drug labels carefully: the drug concentration is expressed as the dose strength contained in a volume of solution.
■ Dilute powders with the appropriate diluent (usually tap water).
■ Measure oral solutions with a medicine cup, dropper, or syringe.

Calculating with different systems

■ First, find the standard equivalent value with a conversion table.
■ Then calculate the dosage using the ratio and proportion method.
■ The standard equivalent values equal the unknown quantity over the quantity ordered.

Desired-over-have method

■ The amount desired over the amount you have equals the equivalent amount desired over the equivalent amount you have.
■ For both fractions, verify that the units of measure in the numerators and denominators correspond to one another.

Transdermal patches

■ Transdermal patch drugs penetrate the outer layers of the skin by passive diffusion and then are absorbed into the circulation.
■ These drugs have a slow onset of action, so it may take hours or even days to achieve a therapeutic drug level.

Topical drug calculations

■ Use your own judgment in accordance with the practitioner's general instructions.
■ Follow specific guidelines for drugs prescribed for a systemic effect.

Rectal drug calculations

■ Use the proportion method with ratios or fractions.
■ A dose is typically prescribed to be provided in one suppository (occasionally two).

◼️◼️ Hit or miss

Label each statement with a "T" for "True" or an "F" for "False."

____ 1. Drugs that are administered orally are never in liquid form.

____ 2. Most oral drugs are available in a limited number of strengths or concentrations.

____ 3. The ability to calculate prescribed dosages isn't essential to nursing.

____ 4. Before you can administer an oral drug safely, you must make sure that it's the correct drug and the correct dosage.

____ 5. When you read the drug label, you should note its expiration date.

____ 6. If the drug has two names, the generic name typically appears in uppercase print.

____ 7. The generic name is a simplified form of the drug's chemical name.

> Surfing through patient care is easy when you know your oral drug basics!

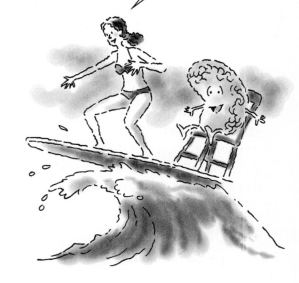

◼️◼️ Finish line

List the various components of each part of the drug label.

1. _____

Each 5 mL (1 teaspoonful) contains sugar and spice 40 mg, everything nice 200 mg, alcohol 0.26% and addedd as preservatives methylparaben 0.1%, sodium benzoate 0.1%.

For indications, dosage, precautions, etc., see accompanying package insert.

Store at 15°25°C (59°77°F)

SHAKE WELL BEFORE USING
Dispose in tight, light-resistant container as defined in the USP.

Manufactured for Fruit Pharmaceutical, Anywhere, PA 12345
By:
BigFruit Pharmaceutical, Anywhere, NJ 67891

REV.6/98
0987654

MEGA® CHERRY
Suspension
sugar and spice
and everything nice

CHERRY FLAVOR

R̲x Only

1 pint (473 mL)

Fruit Pharmaceutical

2. _____

3. _____

4. _____

5. _____

6. _____

7. _____

■ Finish line

Take these crunched versions of practitioners' drug orders and stretch them out into their full instruction form.

1. FeSO$_4$ 325 mg P.O. t.i.d. a.c.

_____

_____

2. Procardia 10 mg P.O. t.i.d. & prn SBP greater than 180

_____

_____

3. oxacillin 1 g IVPB q 6 h × 24 hours

_____

_____

4. D$_5$LR I.V. at 100 ml/h

_____

_____

5. Chloroptic solution 0.5% 2 gtt O.D. Q6°

_____

_____

■ Dosage drills

Test your math skills with this drill.

Be sure to show
how you arrive at
your answer.

A patient has been taking 0.5 g tablets of acetaminophen (Tylenol) P.O. for postoperative pain after an inguinal hernia repair. If the patient took a total of 1,500 mg in 72 hours, how many 0.5 g tablets were taken?

Your answer: _____

Batter's box

Fill in the blanks with the correct information regarding drug error information.

ome oral medications contain _____ drugs. _____ may appear
₁   ₂

fter the drug name. Oral medications are ordered by the _____ name. A drug
₃

as only one _____ name, but it may have _____ trade names.
₄   ₅

he generic drug _____ goes by the trade names Valium and Diastat. U.S.P. is
₆

ne of the legally recognized _____ for drugs.
₇

Options

A. trade

B. N.F.

C. two

D. standards

E. several

F. generic

G. diazepam

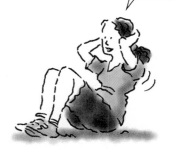

Feel the burn as you learn more oral drug facts!

Pep talk

The study of error is not only in the highest degree prophylactic, but it serves as a stimulating introduction to the study of truth.

—Walter Lippmann

Out of bounds

How is the label on the right different from the label on the left? Circle the differences.

AUGMENTIN®
00mg/5mL

200mg/5mL
NDC 0029-6087-51

Directions for mixing: Tap
ottle until all powder flows
eely. Add approximately 2/3 of
tal water for reconstitution
total = 95 mL); shake
gorously to wet powder. Add
emaining water; again shake
gorously.
osage: Administer every
2 hours. See accompanying
rescribing information.
henylketonurics: Contains
henylalanine 7 mg per 5 mL.

AUGMENTIN®

AMOXICILLIN/
CLAVULANATE
POTASSIUM

FOR ORAL SUSPENSION

When reconstituted, each 5 mL contains:
AMOXICILLIN, 200 MG,
as the trihydrate
CLAVULANIC ACID, 28.5 MG,
as clavulanate potassium

100mL *(when reconstituted)*

Use only if inner seal is intact.
Net contents: Equivalent to 4 g amoxicillin
and 0.57 g clavulanic acid.
Store dry powder at or below 25°C (77°F).

GlaxoSmithKline
Research Triangle Park, NC 27709

3 0029-6087-51 9

LOT

EXP.

eep tightly closed.
hake well before using.
ust be refrigerated.
iscard after 10 days.

gsk GlaxoSmithKline   ℞ only   9405728-H

AUGMENTIN®
400mg/5mL

400mg/5mL
NDC 0029-6092-51

Directions for mixing: Tap
bottle until all powder flows
freely. Add approximately 2/3 of
total water for reconstitution
(total = 90 mL); shake
vigorously to wet powder. Add
remaining water; again shake
vigorously.
Dosage: Administer every
12 hours. See accompanying
prescribing information.
Phenylketonurics: Contains
phenylalanine 7 mg per 5 mL.

AUGMENTIN®

AMOXICILLIN/
CLAVULANATE
POTASSIUM

FOR ORAL SUSPENSION

When reconstituted, each 5 mL contains:
AMOXICILLIN, 400 MG,
as the trihydrate
CLAVULANIC ACID, 57 MG,
as clavulanate potassium

100mL *(when reconstituted)*

Use only if inner seal is intact.
Net contents: Equivalent to 8 g amoxicillin
and 1.14 g clavulanic acid.
Store dry powder at or below 25°C (77°F).

GlaxoSmithKline
Research Triangle Park, NC 27709

3 0029-6092-51 3

LOT

EXP.

**Keep tightly closed.
Shake well before using.
Must be refrigerated.
Discard after 10 days.**

gsk GlaxoSmithKline   ℞ only   9405832-H

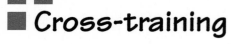

■ Cross-training

Here's an exercise to help pump up your knowledge of oral drug dosages.

Across

3. Cut this type of tablet only in half.

4. Type of chart that helps you convert an analgesic dose from the parenteral route to the oral route

6. Another way to describe a drug's trade name

8. Most dosage calculations require more than one equation, thus requiring you to _____ from one system to another.

Down

1. What's used to change a powder drug to liquid form

2. Strength, in dosage terms

5. Abbreviation for one legally recognized standard of drugs

7. Type of system that provides prepackaged drugs in single-dose containers

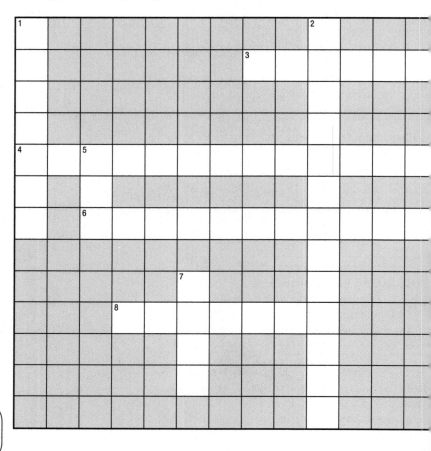

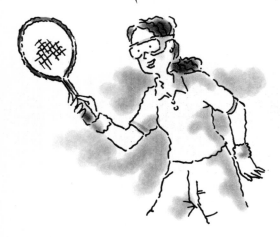

You're hitting these oral drug dosages really hard now!

Starting lineup

The practitioner has ordered 10 mg metoclopramide (Reglan) P.O. b.i.d. a.c. for your patient. Put these steps in the order in which you should proceed before giving an oral drug.

If the drug is supplied in bulk or in a stock bottle, transfer one tablet from the supply to a medication container, pouring from the supply to the lid and then into a container without handling the tablet.	
Place the labeled drug next to the transcribed order on the administration record and carefully compare each part of the label to the order.	
Open the patient's medication drawer, find the drug labeled metoclopraminde (Reglan) 10 mg and note that it's in oral tablet form.	
Go to the patient's bedside, check his identification bracelet, and do your third drug check, comparing the label to the order and checking the administration time again. Then give the drug.	
If the drug comes in a unit-dose packet, don't remove it from the packet until you're at the patient's bedside and ready to administer it. Then do your third drug check. Remove the drug from the packet and give it to the patient, using the packet label for comparison when recording your administration information.	
Before returning the supply to the drawer or shelf, once again compare the label to the order on the administration record, and note whether this is the right administration time.	

▪▪ ▪ Dosage drills

Test your math skills with this drill.

> A practitioner orders 200 mg P.O. of chloral hydrate in liquid form for a patient the night before surgery. The bottle is labeled 500 mg/5 ml. How many milliliters should be prepared?

Be sure to show how you arrive at your answer.

Your answer: _____

▪▪ ▪ Hit or miss

Label each statement with a "T" for "True" or an "F" for "False."

_____ 1. Using the unit-dose drug distribution system can save time.

_____ 2. The unit-dose drug distribution system provides the exact dose of medication needed for each patient.

_____ 3. In the unit-dose system, the nurse computes the number of tablets and prepares the proper dose for administration.

_____ 4. Every facility uses the unit-dose system.

You're soaring for a slam dunk with your knowledge of unit-dose packaging!

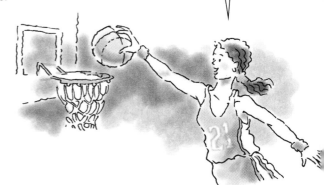

Batter's box

Fill in the blanks with the correct information regarding delivery drug doses.

Pediatric, geriatric, or critical care patients require _____ medications that

₁

may be unusually large or small. Some patients need dosages that are calculated to the near-

est _____ instead of the nearest 10 mg. Some people can't handle drugs that

₂

are delivered by the usual route because their ability to _____ , distribute,

₃

_____ , or excrete drugs is impaired. Other patients who need individualized

₄

dosages include those with conditions that cause _____ drug distribution from

₅

the GI tract or from _____ administration sites to the sites of action.

₆

Options:
A. absorb
B. parenteral
C. abnormal
D. individualized
E. metabolize
F. milligram

Dosage drills

Test your math skills with this drill.

Be sure to show
how you arrive at
your answer.

A practitioner orders 25 g of lactulose (Cephulac) for a patient entering a prehepatic coma. The bottle is labeled 10 g/15 ml. How many milliliters should the patient receive?

Your answer: _____

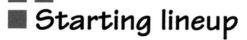

Starting lineup

A patient is scheduled to receive 0.05 mg levothyroxine P.O., but the only drug on hand is in tablets that contain 0.025 mg each. Put the steps below in the order that you would use to figure out how many tablets to give.

0.025 mg : 1 tablet :: 0.05 mg : X

$\dfrac{1\text{ tablet} \times 0.05\text{ mg}}{0.025\text{ mg}} = \dfrac{\cancel{0.025\text{ mg}} \times X}{\cancel{0.025\text{ mg}}}$

1 tablet $\times$ 0.05 mg = 0.025 mg $\times$ X

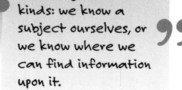

You're kicking out these equations in no time now. Keep going for the goal!

Pep talk

"Knowledge is of two kinds: we know a subject ourselves, or we know where we can find information upon it.

—Samuel Johnson"

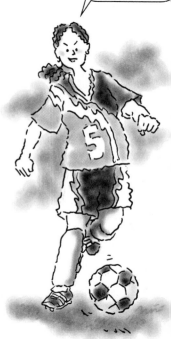

Jumble gym

Unscramble each word to discover the information on the rules for calculating drugs. Then use the circled letters to answer the question below.

Question: **What should you always do with decimals, equations, and units of measure?**

1. R A S M U E E _ _ _ _ ◯ _ _

2. D L M S I E C A ◯ _ _ _ _ _ _ _

3. T O U C A L L A C R ◯ _ _ ◯ _ _ _ _ ◯ _

4. V O E S L _ _ ◯ _ _

5. N M S E A _ ◯ _ _ _

6. M E S E X T E R _ _ _ _ ◯ _ _ _

Answer: _ _ _ B _ _ - _ H _ _ K

Dosage drills

Test your math skills with this drill.

> Be sure to show how you arrive at your answer.

> A practitioner writes an order for propantheline 30 mg by mouth at bedtime for a patient with an ulcer. The only available tablets are 7.5 mg each. How many tablets should be administered?

Your answer: _____

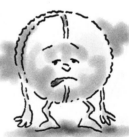

> You mean I'm not already the correct dose? I'm crushed! (Or, I will be soon!)

Hit or miss

Label each statement with a "T" for "True" or an "F" for "False."

_____ 1. Most tablets, capsules, and similar dose forms are available in many different strengths.

_____ 2. Usually you'll administer one tablet or one-half of a scored tablet.

_____ 3. Breaking a scored tablet in portions smaller than one-half usually creates inaccurate doses.

_____ 4. If a dose smaller than one-half of a scored tablet or any portion of an unscored tablet is needed, you shouldn't substitute a commercially available solution.

_____ 5. You can ask the pharmacist to crush the tablet and measure an exact dose.

_____ 6. Some oral preparations shouldn't be opened, broken, scored, or crushed because those actions change the drug's effect.

■ Hit or miss

Is this statement true or false? Label it with a "T" for "True" or an "F" for "False."

Question: **Every dose on the equianalgesic chart provides an equivalent amount of pain control, and any change in medication requires a practitioner's order.**

Answer: _____

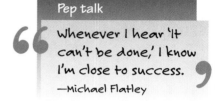
■ Batter's box

Fill in the blanks with the correct information regarding tablet and capsule precautions.

1. Before you break or crush a tablet or capsule, call the _____ to see if the drug is available in smaller dose strengths.

2. Check your drug _____ or check with the pharmacist to see if altering the drug will affect its action.

3. _____-release drugs shouldn't be broken or crushed.

4. Capsules that contain tiny _____ of medication shouldn't be broken or crushed, although you can empty the contents of some of these capsules.

5. _____-coated tablets have a hard coating and shouldn't be crushed.

6. Buccal and _____ tablets shouldn't be crushed.

7. If you need to crush a tablet, use a _____ form.

8. The easiest method is to crush the tablet while it's still in its _____ .

> **Options**
>
> A. sustained
>
> B. package
>
> C. sublingual
>
> D. pharmacist
>
> E. enteric
>
> F. chewable
>
> G. handbook
>
> H. beads

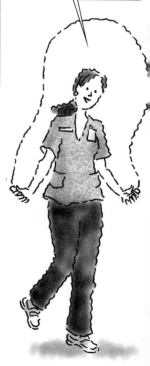

Keep your cardio up by learning the safe ways to administer tablets and capsules!

Jumble gym

Using which type of number relationship can help you determine the amount of tablets, liquids, or injectables needed for administration? Arrange the underlined letters to form the answer.

Walking is <u>o</u>ne of the g<u>r</u>eatest way<u>s</u> to exer<u>ci</u>se. Walk a<u>r</u>ound the block, t<u>o</u> the local <u>p</u>ark or eve<u>n</u> ar<u>o</u>und the sho<u>p</u>ping mall.

Answer: __ __ __ __ __ __ __ __ __ __ __

Dosage drills

Test your math skills with this drill.

Be sure to show how you arrive at your answer.

A practitioner orders 0.125 mg of digoxin (Lanoxin) elixir for a patient developing heart failure and pulmonary edema. The bottle is labeled 0.05 mg/ml. How many milliliters should the nurse administer?

Your answer: _____

Dosage drills

Test your math skills with this drill.

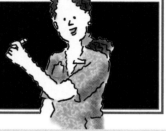

Be sure to show how you arrive at your answer.

> A nurse is to administer 100 mg P.O. of furosemide (Lasix) to a patient returning from surgery with fluid overload. The tablets are each 40 mg. How many tablets should the nurse administer?

Your answer: _____

Starting lineup

Keep treading your way through these dosage drills!

Your patient is receiving 500 mg of cefaclor in an oral suspension. The label reads *250 mg/5 ml,* and the bottle contains 100 ml. Order these steps to figure out how many milliliters of the drug you should give.

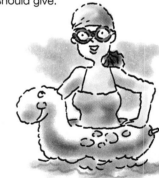

$X = \dfrac{2{,}500 \text{ ml}}{250}$	
$\dfrac{X}{500 \text{ mg}}$	
$\dfrac{X}{500 \text{ mg}} = \dfrac{5 \text{ ml}}{250 \text{ mg}}$	
$\dfrac{5 \text{ ml}}{250 \text{ mg}}$	
$\dfrac{X \times 250 \text{ mg}}{250 \text{ mg}} = \dfrac{5 \text{ ml} \times 500 \text{ mg}}{250 \text{ mg}}$	
$X = 10 \text{ ml}$	
$X \times 250 \text{ mg} = 5 \text{ ml} \times 500 \text{ mg}$	

■■ ■ Batter's box

Fill in the blanks with the correct information regarding the steps needed to perform two-step calculations.

1. Most dosage calculations require more than one _____ .

2. In many cases, you'll need to convert from one measurement _____ to another before determining the amount of medication to administer.

3. To convert between two measurement systems, use a _____ chart to find the standard equivalent value.

4. After using a chart to find standard equivalents, use the ratio-and-proportion or _____ method to calculate the correct dose.

5. Put the standard _____ values in the first ratio or fraction, and put the quantity ordered and the unknown quantity in the second ratio or fraction.

> **Options**
> A. equivalent
> B. system
> C. equation
> D. conversion
> E. fraction

> Who's up for some conversion questions? I can't hear you!

■■ ■ Dosage drills

Test your math skills with this drill.

> Be sure to show how you arrive at your answer.

> A patient must receive 15 ml of potassium chloride four times a day for hypokalemia. The bottle is labeled 40 mEq/30 ml. How many milliequivalents should the nurse give to the patient for each dose?

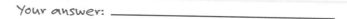

Your answer: _____

■ ■
■ Dosage drills

Test your math skills with this drill.

> Be sure to show how you arrive at your answer.

A practitioner orders amiodarone (Cordarone) for a patient experiencing arrhythmias. The practitioner orders a loading dose of 600 mg. The tablets are marked 200 mg. How many tablets should the nurse administer for the loading dose?

Your answer: _____

■ ■
■ Hit or miss

> Don't lose steam now! Keep going with more information on oral solutions!

Label each statement with a "T" for "True" or an "F" for "False."

_____ 1. Medicine cups are calibrated to measure oral solutions in milliliters, tablespoons, teaspoons, drams, and ounces.

_____ 2. You should hold the cup above eye level for accuracy while pouring an oral solution.

_____ 3. You should hold an oral solution with the medication label turned away from the palm of your hand so that the solution doesn't drip over the label when poured.

_____ 4. Drugs prescribed in drops are usually packaged with a dropper.

_____ 5. Standard droppers shouldn't be used to measure oral solutions in milliliters or teaspoons.

_____ 6. You should never use a syringe to administer an oral drug.

_____ 7. If you leave the plastic tip on a syringe by mistake, the patient can swallow or aspirate it.

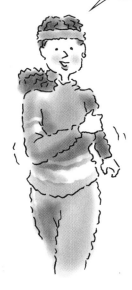

Dosage drills

Test your math skills with this drill.

> Be sure to show how you arrive at your answer.

A practitioner orders 10 mg of propranolol (Inderal) every 6 hours p.r.n. for a patient with hypertension. The bottle of oral solution is labeled 4 mg/ml. How many milliliters should be administered for each dose?

Your answer: _____

Pep talk

"All which is beautiful and noble is the result of reason and calculation."
—Charles Baudelaire

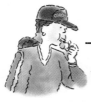

Coaching session

When you need a new measure

To determine a dose when you must first convert to a different measurement system, remember to:
- read the drug order thoroughly, paying close attention to decimal places and zeros
- convert the dose from the system in which it's ordered to the system in which it's available
- calculate the number of capsules or tablets or the amount of solution needed to obtain the desired dose.

Match point

Your patient's drug order, written in apothecaries' units, reads *aspirin gr x̄ P.O. daily*, but the unit-dose package says *aspirin 325 mg*. Match the steps needed to figure out how many tablets you should administer daily with their numerical equivalent

Clues

1. Set up the first fraction with the milligram equivalent of 1 gr. _____

2. Set up the second fraction with the unknown quantity in the appropriate position. _____

3. Set up a proportion with these two fractions. _____

4. Cross-multiply these fractions to set up an equation. _____

5. Divide both sides by 1 gr and cancel units that appear in the numerator and the denominator. _____

6. Determine the number of tables to give by setting up a proportion. _____

7. Cross-multiply the fractions. _____

8. Divide each side of the equation by 325 mg and cancel units that appear in the numerator and the denominator. _____

9. Round your answer. _____

Options

A. $\dfrac{60 \text{ mg}}{1 \text{ grain}} = \dfrac{X}{10 \text{ grains}}$

B. $\dfrac{60 \text{ mg}}{1 \text{ grain}}$

C. $X = 1\frac{4}{5} \text{ tablets} = 2 \text{ tablets}$

D. $X \times 325 \text{ mg} = 1 \text{ tablet} \times 600 \text{ mg}$

E. $60 \text{ mg} \times 10 \text{ grains} = X \times 1 \text{ grain}$

F. $\dfrac{60 \text{ mg} \times 10 \text{ \sout{grains}}}{1 \text{ \sout{grain}}} = \dfrac{X \times 1 \text{ \sout{grain}}}{1 \text{ \sout{grain}}} = X = 600 \text{ m}$

G. $\dfrac{X \times \sout{325 \text{ mg}}}{\sout{325 \text{ mg}}} = \dfrac{1 \text{ tablet} \times 600 \text{ \sout{mg}}}{325 \text{ \sout{mg}}} = \dfrac{600 \text{ tablets}}{325}$

H. $\dfrac{X}{10 \text{ grains}}$

I. $\dfrac{X}{600 \text{ mg}} = \dfrac{1 \text{ tablet}}{325 \text{ mg}}$

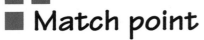

Dosage drills

Test your math skills with this drill.

> A practitioner orders 300,000 units of nystatin suspension (Mycostatin) daily in divided doses for a patient with oral thrush. The drug comes from the pharmacy labeled 5 ml is equal to 500,000 units. How many milliliters should the nurse administer each day?

Be sure to show how you arrive at your answer.

Your answer: _____

Dosage drills

Test your math skills with this drill.

> Be sure to show how you arrive at your answer.

A practitioner orders 2 g of sulfamethoxazole. How many milliliters should be given if the bottle of oral suspension is labeled 500 mg/5ml?

Your answer: _____

Pep talk

" I would study, I would know, I would admire forever. "

—Ralph Waldo Emerson

> Way to p-lunge into two-step calculations!

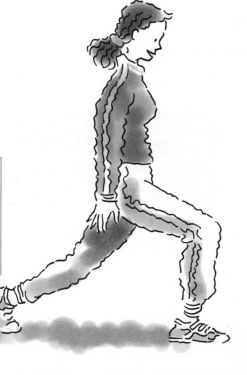

Batter's box

Fill in the blanks with the correct information regarding the desired-over-have method of solving two-step equations.

The desired-over-have method uses _____ to express the known and unknown quantities in proportions.

Make sure the units of _____ used in the numerator and denominator of the first fraction correspond to the units and denominator in the second fraction.

List the amount _____ /amount you have and make that equal to the equivalent amount desired/equivalent amount you have.

Options

A. desired

B. fractions

C. measure

▪▪ ▪ Starting lineup

A drug order calls for 45 mg of magnesium hydroxide (Milk of Magnesia) as a one-time dose, but the only solution on hand contains 30 mg/15 ml. Put these steps in the order needed to figure out how many tablespoons you should give the patient

Cross-multiply the fractions.	
Solve for *X* by dividing each side of the equation by 30 mg and canceling units that appear in both the numerator and denominator.	
Convert the milliliters to tablespoons by using a conversion table.	
Set up the second fraction with the unknown amount desired (*X*) in the appropriate position.	
Set up the first fraction with the amount desired over the amount you have.	
Put the fractions into a proportion.	

▪▪ ▪ Dosage drills

Test your math skills with this drill.

> Be sure to show how you arrive at your answer.

An order is written for propranolol 50 mg P.O., but the only available form is 20mg tablets. How many tablets must the nurse administer?

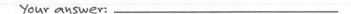

Your answer: _____

Match point

To solve the equation, match the steps in Column 1 with the steps in Column 2.

The drug order reads *digoxin elixir 0.125 mg P.O. stat.* The pharmacy sends you Digoxin 0.5 mg/5 ml. How many milliliters should you give the patient?

Clues

1. Step 1 _____
2. Step 2 _____
3. Step 3 _____
4. Step 4 _____
5. Step 5 _____

Options

A. Cross-multiply the fractions.

B. Set up the first fraction with the amount desired over the amount you have.

C. Set up the second fraction with the unknown amount desired in the appropriate position.

D. Put the fractions into a proportion.

E. Solve for X by dividing both sides of the equation by 0.5 mg.

Dosage drills

Test your math skills with this drill.

Be sure to show how you arrive at your answer.

A practitioner orders 500 mg of amoxicillin (Amoxil) P.O. every 12 hours for a patient with bronchitis. The bottle of oral suspension is labeled 125 mg/5 ml. How many milliliters should the nurse administer for a single dose?

Your answer: _____

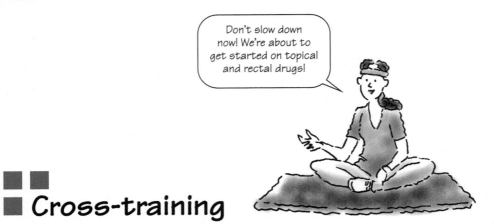

■■ ■ Cross-training

Test your knowledge of topical and rectal drugs and their labels.

Across

2. A synonym for *topical*

4. Rectal drugs include _____ and suppositories.

5. Patients may not be able to take oral drugs because they have this type of tube.

7. Topical drugs are absorbed through the epidermis into this.

8. The first type of name that appears on a topical or rectal drug label

9. Along with creams, lotions, and ointments, these are commonly used for dermatologic treatment or wound care.

Down

1. Type of special instructions that may appear on a topical or rectal drug label

3. Topical drug type used to manage chronic pain

6. Alternate drug route for patients who can't take drugs orally

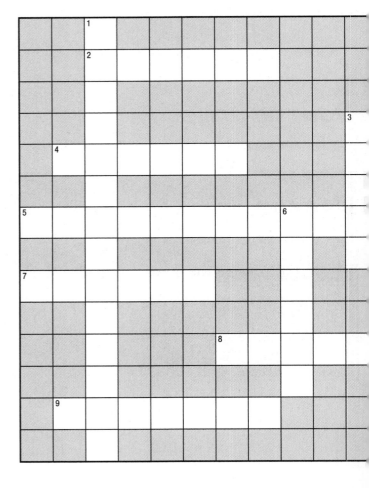

Finish line

Fill in the parts of this topical ointment label.

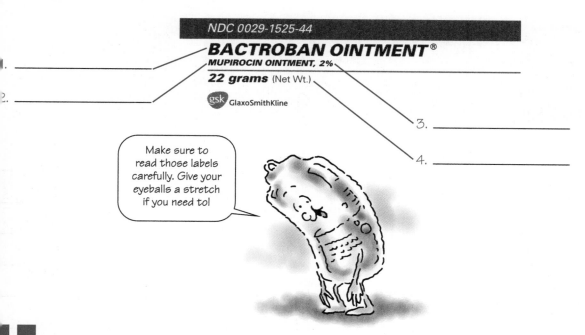

1. _____

2. _____

NDC 0029-1525-44

BACTROBAN OINTMENT®
MUPIROCIN OINTMENT, 2%
22 grams (Net Wt.)

gsk GlaxoSmithKline

3. _____

4. _____

Make sure to read those labels carefully. Give your eyeballs a stretch if you need to!

Dosage drills

Test your math skills with this drill.

Be sure to show how you arrive at your answer.

The practitioner writes an order for lithium carbonate grXX P.O. t.i.d. The drug label states Lithium carbonate USP 300 mg/capsule. How many capsules should the nurse give to the patient for one dose?

Your answer: _____

■ Dosage drills

Test your math skills with this drill.

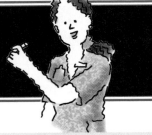

Be sure to show how you arrive at your answer.

> How many teaspoons of a 325 mg/5 ml elixir would a nurse give to deliver 650 mg of acetaminophen?

Your answer: _____

■ Hit or miss

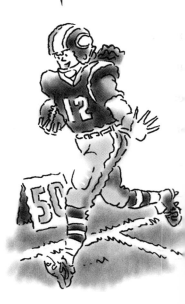

Stay strong as you tackle patches!

Label each statement with a "T" for "True" or an "F" for "False."

_____ 1. In the past, topical drugs were used almost solely for their local effects.

_____ 2. Today, topical drugs are still only used for their local effects.

_____ 3. Transdermal patch drugs aren't absorbed into the circulation.

_____ 4. Transdermal patch drugs penetrate the outer layers of the skin by way of passive diffusion at a constant rate.

_____ 5. Patches are a good way to administer drugs that aren't absorbed well in the GI tract and those that are eliminated too quickly to be effective.

_____ 6. Patches can't maintain consistent blood levels of a drug.

_____ 7. Patches have a slow onset of action.

_____ 8. Reversing the toxic effects of patches is relatively easy.

Dosage drills

Test your math skills with this drill.

> A patient is to receive 0.25 mg of Synthroid. The medication is only available in tablets that contain 125 mcg each. How many tablets should the nurse administer?

Be sure to show how you arrive at your answer.

Your answer: _____

Batter's box

Fill in the blanks with the correct information regarding combination product alerts.

pical _____ may contain more
                    1

an one _____ . For example,
                    2

citracin Plus ointment contains bacitracin,

omycin, polymyxin B, and

_____ . Carefully note all
        3

_____ when checking labels and
        4

ke sure that your patient isn't

_____ to any of them.
        5

Options

A. drug

B. lidocaine

C. preparations

D. allergic

E. ingredients

Now let's hit 'em with a one-two combination— combination products!

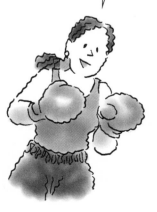

Match point

Match the patches in the first column with their trade names in the second column.

Clues

1. Nitroglycerin _____
2. Estradiol _____
3. Testosterone _____
4. Clonidine _____
5. Nicotine _____
6. Fentanyl _____

Options

A. Catapres TTS
B. Androderm
C. Duragesic
D. Climara
E. Habitrol
F. Nitro-Dur

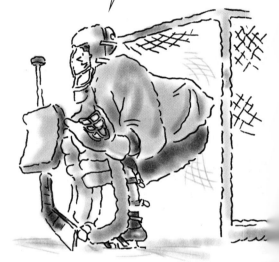

> Getting checked is a good thing when it comes to patches.

Strikeout

Strike out the incorrect statements.

1. The Testoderm patch is applied once daily to clean, hairless scrotal skin.

2. Scopolamine is used to treat nausea, vomiting, and vertigo.

3. Habitrol, Nicoderm, Nicotrol, and ProStep should be used without other therapy.

4. Transdermal fentanyl is administered to treat hypertension.

5. Transdermal estradiol is administered on an intermittent cyclic schedule.

6. A new transdermal nitroglycerin patch is applied daily and removed after 12 to 14 hours to prevent the patient from developing a tolerance to the drug.

7. The clonidine patch is used to treat hypotension.

Pep talk

Constant attention by a good nurse may be just as important as a major operation by a surgeon.

—Dag Hammarskjöld

Jumble gym

Unscramble the terms relating to transdermal patches to answer the question below.

Question: Transdermal patches must be checked frequently because they can become what?

1. A B I P R O T O N S _ _ O _ _ _ _ O _ _

2. P A P L Y _ _ O _ _

3. L O B D O _ _ _ _ O

4. C A L L O _ _ O _ _

5. T S E N O _ _ _ O _

6. A R E C L E N T O _ _ O _ _ _ _ _ _

7. M A N D R E L T S A R _ _ O _ _ O _ _ _ _ _

Answer: _ _ _ _ _ _ _ _ _ _

Your grip on this topic sure isn't patchy!

Dosage drills

Test your math skills with this drill.

Be sure to show how you arrive at your answer.

The practitioner orders a 650 mg aspirin suppository for a patient. The pharmacy is closed and the only aspirin on hand contains 325 mg per suppository. How many suppositories should you give?

Your answer: _____

Dosage drills

Test your math skills with this drill.

> Be sure to show how you arrive at your answer.

A practitioner orders ibuprofen 800 mg P.O. every 6 hours, but only 400 mg tablets are available. How many tablets should the nurse administer?

Your answer: _____

Batter's box

> Catch and release! As in, catch up on information about drug release!

Fill in the blanks with the correct information regarding drug release.

1. Drug _____ in transdermal patches vary depending on the _____ of the patch.

2. The drug's concentration isn't as important as its rate of _____ .

3. Two patches containing the same drug in different concentrations may actually release the same _____ of drug per hour.

Options

A. design

B. amount

C. release

D. concentrations

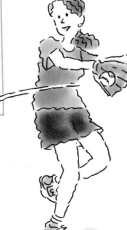

Dosage drills

Test your math skills with this drill.

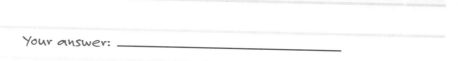

Be sure to show
how you arrive at
your answer.

A practitioner orders bisacodyl suppository 10 mg p.r.n. The
only available dosage is 5 mg per suppository. How many
suppositories should the nurse administer?

Your answer: _____

Match point

Keep swinging
away at this rectal
drug dosage drill!

Match the type of patch to its characteristics. (Note that
some answers will be used more than once.)

Clues

1. Can prevent angina _____

2. Held in a reservoir behind a membrane
that allows controlled drug absorption
through the skin _____

3. Can control nausea _____

4. Is available in doses of 25, 50, 75, and
100 mcg/hour _____

5. Can manage chronic pain _____

6. Should be changed every 72 hours _____

Options

A. Fentanyl

B. Nitroglycerin

C. Clonidine

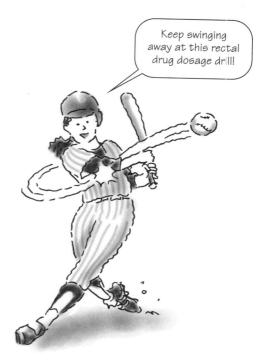

■ Hit or miss

Label each statement with a "T" for "True" or an "F" for "False."

_____ 1. Transdermal patches are changed at random intervals.

_____ 2. To apply a new patch, you should put it on top of the old patch at the appropriate time.

_____ 3. When applying ointment from a tube, you should estimate the dose using your best judgment.

■ Batter's box

Fill in the blanks with the correct information regarding ointment application.

When the practitioner prescribes an _____ as part of wound care or
            1

dermatologic treatment, he usually leaves the _____ to apply up to
                                              2

_____ . He may give general guidance, such as "use a
       3

_____ layer" or "apply thickly." When an ointment contains a drug
       4

intended for a _____ effect, more _____ administration
                      5   6

guidelines are necessary. Many ointments, including nitroglycerin, are available in

_____ .
       7

Options:

A. specific

B. thin

C. systemic

D. tubes

E. you

F. ointment

G. amount

Squeeze these ointment facts into your studying!

Dosage drills

Test your math skills with this drill.

Be sure to show how you arrive at your answer.

A practitioner orders the laxative psyllium at a dose of 1 g P.O. daily for a patient after a fecal impaction has been removed. Available tablets are 500 mg each. How many tablets should the nurse administer to the patient each day?

Your answer: _____

Finish line

The practitioner has ordered 1.5 inches of nitroglycerin ointment for a patient's wound care. On the paper ruler illustration below, draw the line to where you would measure out the amount of ointment.

Keep plowing through! Rectal drug dosages are the last hill to climb!

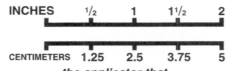

NITRO-BID®
(Nitroglycerin Ointment USP, 2%)

INCHES	½	1	1½	2

CENTIMETERS	1.25	2.5	3.75	5

the applicator that measures the dose
E. FOUGERA & CO.
a division of Altana Inc.
MELVILLE, NEW YORK 11747

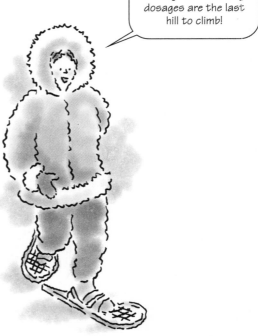

■ Hit or miss

Label each statement with a "T" for "True" or an "F" for "False."

_____ 1. Rectal drugs include enemas and suppositories.

_____ 2. To calculate the number of suppositories to give, you should use the proportion method with ratios or fractions.

_____ 3. The practitioner rarely prescribes drugs in the dose provided by one suppository.

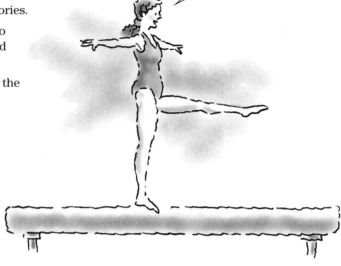

Now, let's balance your book knowledge with some real-world application!

■ Starting lineup

Your pediatric patient needs 120 mg of acetaminophen by suppository. The package label reads *acetaminophen suppositories 60 mg.* Put these steps in the order needed to figure out how many suppositories you should give the patient.

Cross-multiply the fractions.

Solve for *X* by dividing each side of the equation by 60 mg and canceling units that appear in both the numerator and denominator.

Set up the second fraction with the desired dose and the unknown number of suppositories.

Set up the first fraction with the known suppository dose.

Put the first and second fractions into a proportion.

Dosage drills

Test your math skills with this drill.

> Be sure to show how you arrive at your answer.

A nurse must administer 400 mg of dyphylline every 12 hours to a patient with emphysema. The bottle of oral elixir is labeled 100 mg/15 ml. How many milliliters should the nurse administer in each dose?

Your answer: _____

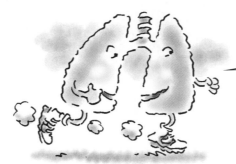

> You're giving these dosage drills a run for their money!

Hit or miss

Is the following equation answer true or false? Label it with a "T" for "True" or an "F" for "False."

Question: The practitioner orders a 100-mg Tigan suppository for your patient. The pharmacy is closed, and the only Tigan on hand contains 200 mg per suppository. You should give 1 suppository.

Answer: _____

■■
■ Match point

Match the suppository dosage quantity with the instructions for checking a suppository dosage quantity with the quantities themselves.

Clues

1. Check your figures, ask another nurse to check them, then ask the pharmacist whether the drug is available in other dosage strengths. _____

2. Confirm the dose with the practitioner, and check with the pharmacist, who may be able to give you one suppository with an adequate amount of the drug. _____

3. Check your figures, ask another nurse to check them, then ask the pharmacist if the dose is available in one suppository. _____

Options

A. Less than one suppository

B. More than one suppository

C. More than two suppositories

■■
■ Dosage drills

Test your math skills with this drill.

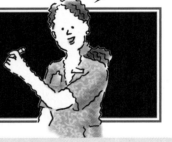

Be sure to show how you arrive at your answer.

> A practitioner orders 750 mg of methocarbamol (Robaxin) P.O. every 8 hours p.r.n. for a patient with muscular back pain. The pharmacy sends tablets labeled 500 mg. How many tablets should the nurse administer?

Your answer: _____

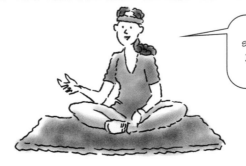

You did well on this section, but you're not done yet. Take a short rest and then keep moving!

5

Calculating parenteral injections

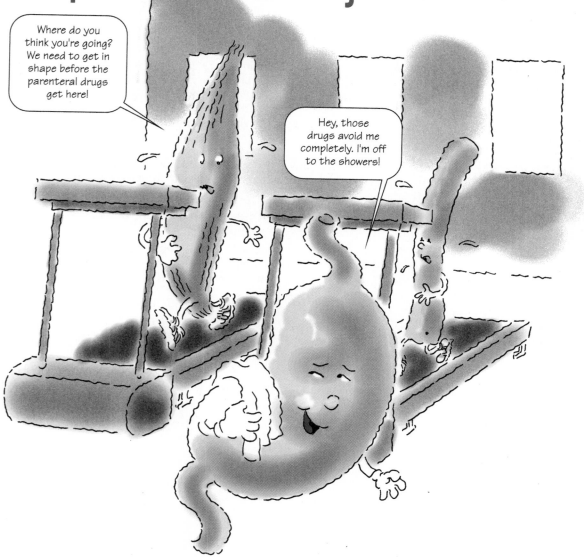

■ Warm-up

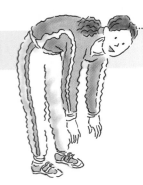

Calculating parenteral injections review

Intradermal injections

■ This route is used to anesthetize the skin for invasive procedures and to test for allergies, tuberculosis, histoplasmosis, and other diseases.
■ Amount of drug injected is less than 0.5 ml.
■ Syringe and needle are a 1-ml syringe with a 25G to 27G needle that's ⅜″ to ⅝″ long.

SubQ injections

■ Drugs commonly given subQ include insulin, heparin, tetanus toxoid, and some opioids.
■ Amount of drug injected is 0.5 to 1 ml.
■ Needle is 23G to 28G and ½″ to ⅝″ long.
■ When injecting insulin or heparin, don't aspirate for blood and don't massage the site.

I.M. injections

■ This route is used for drugs that require quick absorption or those that are irritating to tissue.
■ Amount of drug injected is 0.5 to 3 ml.
■ Needles are 18G to 23G and 1″ to 3″ long.
■ Before injection, aspirate for blood to make sure that the needle isn't in a vein.

Syringe types

■ Standard syringes come in a variety of sizes (3, 5, 10, 20, 30, 50, and 60 ml).
■ Tuberculin syringes (commonly used for intradermal injections) are 1-ml syringes marked to hundredths of a milliliter, allowing for accurate measurement of very small doses.
■ Prefilled syringes—sterile syringes that contain a premeasured drug dose—require a special holder (Carpuject or Tubex) to release the drug from the cartridge.

Needle terminology

■ Gauge: inside diameter of the needle (the smaller the gauge, the larger the diameter)
■ Bevel: angle at which the needle tip is open (may be short, medium, or long)
■ Length: distance from needle tip to hub (ranges from ⅜″ to 3″)

Important parts of a parenteral drug label

■ Trade name
■ Generic name
■ Total volume of solution in the container
■ Dose strength or concentration
■ Approved routes of administration
■ Expiration date
■ Special instructions

Ratio solutions

■ Solute is a drug in liquid or solid form that's added to a solvent (diluent) to make a solution.
■ Solution is a liquid (usually sterile water) containing a dissolved solute.
■ W:V solution: First number represents the amount of drug grams; second number is the volume of finished solution in milliliters.
■ V:V solution: First number is the amount of drug in milliliters; second number is the volume of finished solution in milliliters.

Insulin doses

■ Measured in units
■ Based on drug potency (not weight)
■ Classified by origin (human or animal) and action time
■ Most common (universal) concentration is U-100 insulin

Insulin action times

■ Rapid acting: regular, lispro
■ Intermediate acting: lente; NPH; isophane 70%/regular 30%; isophane 50%/regular 50%
■ Long acting: ultralente, insulin glargine

Powders for reconstitution

■ The fluid volume increases with the added diluent.
■ Single-strength powders are reconstituted to one dose strength per administration route.
■ Multiple-strength powders are reconstituted to appropriate strengths by adjusting the amount of diluent.

Hit or miss

Label each statement with a "T" for "True" or an "F" for "False."

___ 1. The term *parenteral* refers to "outside the intestines."

___ 2. Drugs may be administered parenterally through the skin, subcutaneous tissue, muscle, or vein.

___ 3. Parenteral drugs may be supplied as liquids or powders and they never require reconstitution.

___ 4. You need to perform calculations to determine the amount of liquid medication to inject only when using a liquid parenteral drug.

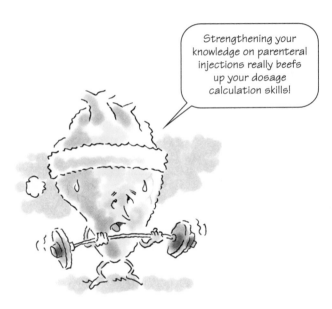

Strengthening your knowledge on parenteral injections really beefs up your dosage calculation skills!

Jumble gym

Unscramble each word to discover three of the four types of injections for parenteral drugs.

L A M T A R D I E R N __ __ __ __ __ __ __ __ __ __ __

S A U T E S N U O B U C __ __ __ __ __ __ __ __ __ __ __ __

C I M N A R S A U R T L U __ __ __ __ __ __ __ __ __ __ __ __ __ __

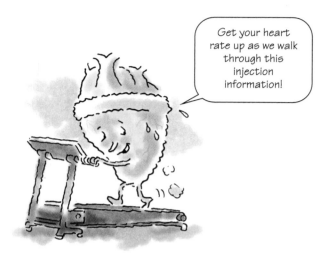

Get your heart rate up as we walk through this injection information!

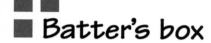

Batter's box

Fill in the blanks with the correct answer options regarding parenteral drugs.

Giving parenteral drugs safely depends on choosing the right type of _____

1

for the patient's _____ and the right _____ and needle for

2   3

the _____ of injection.

4

Options
A. condition
B. injection
C. syringe
D. type

Hit or miss

Label each statement with a "T" for "True" or an "F" for "False."

_____ 1. In an intradermal injection, medication is injected into the dermis.

_____ 2. The dermis is the outermost layer of skin.

_____ 3. An intradermal injection is never used to anesthetize the skin for invasive procedures.

_____ 4. An intradermal injection is used to test for allergies and tuberculosis.

_____ 5. An intradermal injection isn't used to test for histoplasmosis.

Starting lineup

Put these steps in the order needed for the basic procedure to perform an intradermal injection.

Stretch the skin taut with one hand.	
Clean the skin thoroughly.	
Inject the drug.	
Insert the needle quickly at a 10- to 15-degree angle to a depth of about 0.5 cm.	

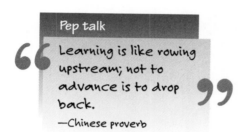

Pep talk

Learning is like rowing upstream; not to advance is to drop back.

—Chinese proverb

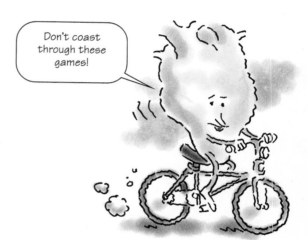

Don't coast through these games!

Batter's box

Fill in the blanks with the correct answer options regarding subcutaneous injection.

a _____ injection, the drug is injected into the
1

ubcutaneous tissue, which is _____ the dermis
2

d above the _____ . Drugs are absorbed
3

_____ in this layer than in the _____
4   5

ecause the subcutaneous layer has more _____ .
6

sulin, _____ , tetanus toxoid, and some opioid
7

algesics are injected through this _____ .
8

Options

A. heparin

B. route

C. beneath

D. subQ

E. muscle

F. faster

G. capillaries

H. dermis

■■ Strikeout

Strike out the incorrect statements.

1. Only 0.5 to 1 ml of a drug can be injected subQ.
2. The needles used for subQ injections are 23G to 28G.
3. The needles used for subQ injections are ¾″ to 1″ long.
4. The lateral areas of the upper arms and thighs are subQ injection sites.
5. The abdomen isn't a subQ injection site.
6. The upper back is a subQ injection site.

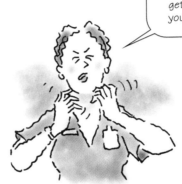

Are these subQ games getting under your skin yet?

■■ Starting lineup

Put these steps in the order needed for the basic procedure to perform a subQ injection.

Administer the injection.	
Pinch the patient's skin between your index finger and thumb and insert the needle.	
Clean the skin.	
Choose the injection site.	
Massage the site (unless you're giving insulin or heparin).	
Aspirate for blood to make sure that the needle isn't in a vein (unless injecting insulin or heparin).	

Cross-training

Here's an exercise to help expand your knowledge of intramuscular injections.

Across

3. The rectus _____ muscle is one I.M. injection site.

5. The instrument used to administer an I.M. injection

6. Any I.M. injection goes into a _____ .

8. I.M. injections are used for drugs that irritate tissues if given by a _____ route.

Down

1. The _____ gluteal muscle is another I.M. injection site.

2. The _____ of I.M. needles is 18G to 23G.

4. An I.M. injection site depends on the patient's muscle _____ .

7. The _____ for I.M. injections ranges from 0.5 to 3 ml.

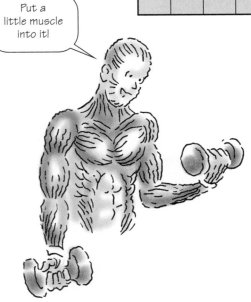

Put a little muscle into it!

Batter's box

Fill in the blanks with the correct answer options regarding the basic procedure for administering intramuscular injections.

1. Choose the _____ site.

2. Clean the _____ .

3. Using a quick, _____ action, insert the needle at a 75- to 90-degree angle.

4. Before injecting the drug, _____ for blood to make sure that the needle isn't in a vein.

5. Push the _____ and keep the syringe steady.

6. After the drug is injected, pull the needle straight out and apply _____ to the site.

> **Options**
> A. aspirate
> B. pressure
> C. injection
> D. skin
> E. plunger
> F. dartlike

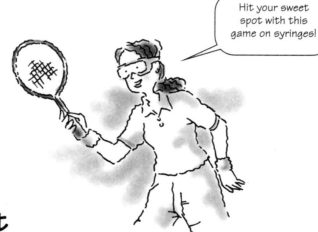

Hit your sweet spot with this game on syringes!

Strikeout

Strike out the incorrect statement.

1. Seven basic types of hypodermic syringes are used to measure and administer parenteral drugs.

2. A standard syringe is a type of hypodermic syringe.

3. Tuberculin and prefilled syringes are types of hypodermic syringes.

4. The drugs that hypodermic syringes are used to measure are ordered in milliliters.

> **Pep talk**
>
> " Flaming enthusiasm, backed up by horse sense and persistence, is the quality that most frequently makes for success.
> —Dale Carnegie "

Hit or miss

Label each statement with a "T" for "True" or an "F" for "False."

_____ 1. Standard syringes are available in 15, 25, 35, 55 and 75 ml.

_____ 2. Each standard syringe consists of a plunger, a barrel, a hub, a needle, and dead space.

_____ 3. The dead space holds the fluid that remains in the syringe and needle after the plunger is partially depressed.

_____ 4. All syringes have dead space.

Strikeout

Strike out the incorrect statements.

1. The calibration marks on a syringe allow you to accurately measure drug doses.

2. The 5-ml syringe is the most commonly used syringe.

3. The 3-ml syringe is calibrated in tenths of a milliliter on the right.

4. The 3-ml syringe has large marks for every 0.5 ml on the right.

5. The large volume syringes are calibrated in 1- to 5-ml increments.

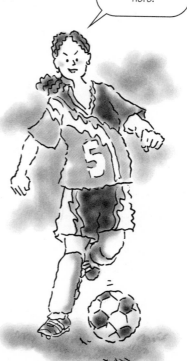

Good measurement is your goal here.

■ Finish line

Label each part of the standard syringe.

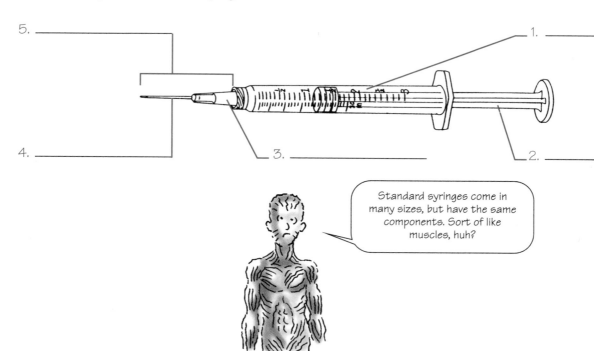

5. _____

4. _____

1. _____

3. _____

2. _____

> Standard syringes come in many sizes, but have the same components. Sort of like muscles, huh?

■ Starting lineup

Put these steps in the order needed to administer a drug via syringe.

Use aseptic technique.
Pull the plunger back until the top ring of the plunger's black portion aligns with the correct calibration mark.
Calculate the dose.
Draw the drug into the syringe.
Administer the drug.
Double-check the dose measurement.

Hit or miss

Label each statement with a "T" for "True" or an "F" for "False."

___ 1. Parenteral drugs come in various dose strengths or concentrations.

___ 2. The usual adult dose of a parenteral drug can be contained in 3 to 6 ml of solution.

___ 3. If a patient needs a dose of a parenteral drug that's larger than 3 ml, you should give it to him in two injections at two different sites.

___ 4. Giving a patient a dose of a parenteral drug that's larger than 3 ml in three injections at three different sites allows for proper drug absorption.

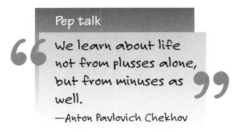

Pep talk

We learn about life not from plusses alone, but from minuses as well.

—Anton Pavlovich Chekhov

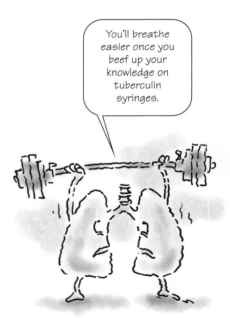

You'll breathe easier once you beef up your knowledge on tuberculin syringes.

Batter's box

Fill in the blanks with the correct answer options regarding tuberculin syringes.

Tuberculin syringes are commonly used for _____ injections. Tuberculin
                                              1

syringes are commonly used to administer _____ amounts of drugs,
                                              2

such as those given to _____ patients or those on intensive care units.
                          3

Each tuberculin syringe is calibrated in _____ of a milliliter on the right,
                                            4

allowing you to accurately administer doses as small as 0.25 ml. Tuberculin syringes

are also marked for alternate _____ of a milliliter.
                                5

Options

A. tenths

B. intradermal

C. hundredths

D. pediatric

E. small

■ Hit or miss

Label each statement with a "T" for "True" or an "F" for "False."

_____ 1. Prefilled syringes usually come with a cartridge-needle unit.

_____ 2. Prefilled syringes require a special holder called a *Carpuject* or *Tubex* to release the drug from the cartridge.

_____ 3. Each prefilled cartridge is calibrated in hundredths of a milliliter and has smaller marks for half and full milliliters.

_____ 4. All of the cartridges for prefilled syringes can only hold one drug.

_____ 5. You can mix more than one drug in a prefilled syringe.

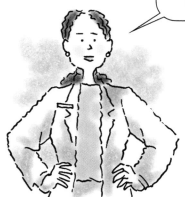

I hope none of your answer blanks are prefilled!

■ Strikeout

Strike out the incorrect statements.

1. Prefilled syringes are labeled with the drug name and dose.

2. An advantage of a prefilled syringe is that you don't have to measure each drug dose.

3. Most manufacturers include the exact amount of a drug in a prefilled syringe.

4. Prefilled syringes are available in all doses.

5. You should carefully document the amount of any drug you discard from a prefilled syringe.

> Time to step things up for this game on closed-system devices!

Finish line

Label each part of the prefilled syringe.

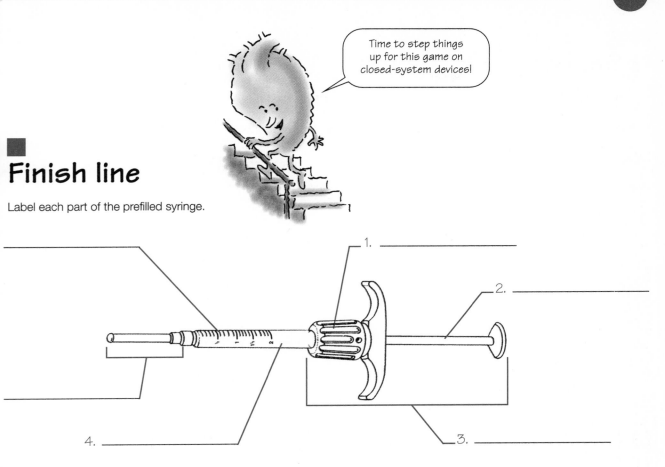

1. _____

2. _____

3. _____

4. _____

Starting lineup

Put these steps in the order needed to prepare a closed-system device.

Flip the protective cap off both ends of the closed-system device.	
Hold the drug chamber in one hand and the syringe and needle in the other.	
Remove the needle cap and expel air and extra medication.	
Insert the drug chamber into the syringe section.	

Batter's box

Fill in the blanks with the correct answers regarding needle terminology.

The needle's _____ refers to the inside diameter of a needle. The smaller the
$\quad\quad\quad\quad\quad$ 1

gauge, the larger the _____ . The needle's _____ refers to the
$\quad\quad\quad\quad\quad$ 2 $\quad\quad\quad\quad\quad\quad\quad\quad\quad\quad$ 3

angle at which the needle tip is opened. The bevel may be short, _____ or long.
$\quad\quad\quad\quad\quad\quad\quad\quad\quad\quad\quad\quad\quad\quad\quad\quad$ 4

The needle's _____ describes the distance from the needle tip to needle hub.
$\quad\quad\quad\quad\quad$ 5

Options

A. diameter

B. bevel

C. gauge

D. medium

E. length

You'll be a pro once you can pick the right needles for your patients!

Match point

Match the type of needle in Column 1 to its characteristics in Column 2.

Clues

1. I.V. needles _____

2. Filter needles _____

3. Intradermal needles _____

4. Subcutaneous needles _____

5. I.M. needles _____

Options

A. $\frac{3}{8}''$ to $\frac{5}{8}''$ long; have short bevels; 25G to 27G in diameter

B. $1\frac{1}{2}''$ long; have medium bevels; 20G in diameter; used for preparing a solution from a vial or ampule

C. 1″ to 3″ long; have medium bevels; 18G to 23G in diameter

D. 1″ to 3″ long; have long bevels; 14G to 25G in diameter

E. $\frac{1}{2}''$ to $\frac{5}{8}''$ long; have medium bevels; 23G to 28G in diameter

Starting lineup

The practitioner prescribes 25 mg of I.M. meperidine q4H for your patient's pain. The drug is available in a prefilled syringe containing 50 mg of morphine/ml. List the steps below that you would use to figure out how many milliliters of morphine you should discard.

$$\frac{25 \text{ mg}}{X}$$

$$\frac{50 \text{ mg}}{1 \text{ ml}}$$

$$0 \text{ mg} \times X = 25 \text{ mg} \times 1 \text{ ml}$$

$$\frac{50 \text{ mg}}{1 \text{ ml}} = \frac{25 \text{ mg}}{X}$$

$$\frac{\cancel{50 \text{ mg}} \times X}{\cancel{50 \text{ mg}}} = \frac{25 \cancel{\text{ mg}} \times 1 \text{ ml}}{50 \cancel{\text{ mg}}}$$

$$X = \frac{25 \text{ ml}}{50}$$

$$X = 0.5 \text{ ml}$$

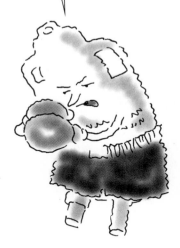

Go ahead and knock out this injection problem!

■ Match point

The practitioner orders 3 mg haloperidol (Haldol) I.M. q4h for your patient with anxiety. The vial contains 5 mg/ml. How much Haldol should you give? To solve the equation, match the steps in Column 1 to the correct equation steps in Column 2.

Clues

1. Step 1 _____
2. Step 2 _____
3. Step 3 _____
4. Step 4 _____
5. Step 5 _____

Options

A. $3 \text{ mg} : X$

B. $3 \text{ mg} \times 1 \text{ ml} = 5 \text{ mg} \times X$

C. $\dfrac{3 \text{ mg} \times 1 \text{ ml}}{5 \text{ mg}} = \dfrac{5 \text{ mg} \times X}{5 \text{ mg}}$

$$\frac{3 \text{ ml}}{5} = X$$

$$X = 0.6 \text{ ml}$$

D. $5 \text{ mg} : 1 \text{ ml} :: 3 \text{ mg} : X$

E. $5 \text{ mg} : 1 \text{ ml}$

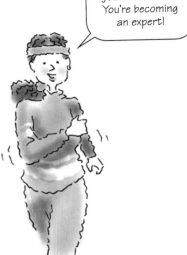

Don't break your stride now. You're becoming an expert!

■ Finish line

Label the parts of the drug label with information you need to know to safely administer a parenteral drug.

1. _____

2. _____

3. _____

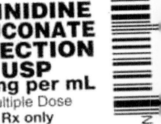

NDC 0002-1407-01
10 mL   VIAL No. 530
℞   *Lilly*
QUINIDINE GLUCONATE INJECTION USP
80 mg per mL
Multiple Dose
Rx only

Starting lineup

The practitioner prescribes 120 mg of furosemide for your patient. The available vial contains 100 mg/ml. Properly order the steps that you would use to figure out how much furosemide you should give.

100 mg : 1 ml	
100 mg : 1 ml :: 120 mg : X	
120 mg : X	
$\dfrac{1\ ml \times 120\ \cancel{mg}}{100\ \cancel{mg}} = \dfrac{100\ \cancel{mg} \times X}{100\ \cancel{mg}}$	
$\dfrac{120\ ml}{100} = X$	
$X = 1.2\ ml$	
1 ml × 120 mg = 100 mg × X	

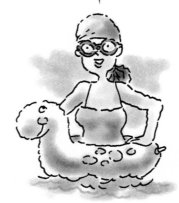

Try not to wash away in all this calculation information!

■■ ■ Hit or miss

Label each statement with a "T" for "True" or an "F" for "False."

_____ 1. On the label of a parenteral solution, you'll see trade name, generic name, total volume of solution in the container, and dose strength or concentration.

_____ 2. On the label of a parenteral solution, you'll see dose strength or concentration, approved routes of administration, and expiration date.

_____ 3. A solute is a liquid form of a drug.

_____ 4. Sterile water is a common diluent.

_____ 5. In normal saline solution, the solvent is the salt and the purified water is the solute.

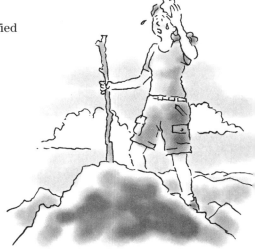

Getting tired? Don't g[ ]up! A solutio[ ]will present itself soon!

■■ ■ Batter's box

Fill in the blanks with the correct answers regarding solution labels.

A solution may be expressed as _____ per volume (W/V) or

volume per _____ (V/V). If the label says 5% _____
      2   3

boric acid solution, the solution contains 5 g of boric acid in 100 ml of finished

solution. If the label says 70% (V/V) isopropyl alcohol, the solution contains 70

_____ of isopropyl alcohol in 100 ml of finished solution. If the
      4

label says _____ (V/V) hydrogen peroxide, the solution contains
      5

2 ml of hydrogen peroxide in 100 ml of finished solution. If the label says 10%

_____ glycerin, the solution contains _____ of
      6   7

glycerin in 100 ml of finished solution.

Options

A. (V/V)

B. (W/V)

C. 2%

D. 10 ml

E. ml

F. volume

G. weight

■■
■ Match point

Match the solution contents in the first column to their corresponding labels in the second column.

ues

1. 10 ml of glycerin in 100 ml of finished solution _____
2. 2 ml of hydrogen peroxide in 100 ml of finished solution _____
3. 1 g of silver nitrate in 100 ml of finished solution _____
4. 1 g of benzalkonium chloride in 750 ml of finished solution _____

Options

A. 1 : 750 (W : V)
B. 1 : 100 (W : V)
C. 2 : 100 (V : V)
D. 10 : 100 (V : V)

■■
■ Hit or miss

Label each statement with a "T" for "True" or an "F" for "False."

____ 1. % = weight/volume = milliliters solute/100 ml finished solution

____ 2. % = volume/volume = grams solute/100 ml finished solution

____ 3. In a weight per volume solution, the first number signifies the amount of drug in grams.

____ 4. In a volume per volume solution, the second number signifies the volume of finished solution in milliliters.

> **Pep talk**
>
> 66 Learning and teaching should not stand on opposite banks and just watch the river flow by; instead, they should embark together on a journey down the water. Through an active, reciprocal exchange, teaching can strengthen learning and how to learn. 99
>
> —Loris Malaguzzi

Cross-training

Here's an exercise to help expand your knowledge of insulin and unit-based drugs.

Across

1. Anticoagulant used to prevent thrombosis and embolism
3. This type of reaction results from an error in insulin calculation or administration.
6. Disease that results from a lack of insulin or from insulin resistance
7. Hormone that regulates carbohydrate metabolism

Down

2. Organ that produces insulin
4. Insulin administration method
5. Method of injection for patient with chronic diabetes
8. This system is based on an international standard of drug potency, not a weight.

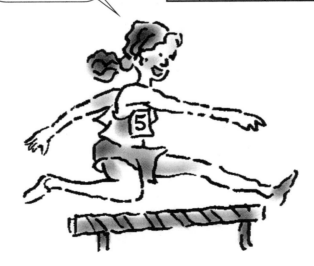

Jump right into this insulin information!

Finish line

Label the parenteral drug that's measured in units with the information shown here.

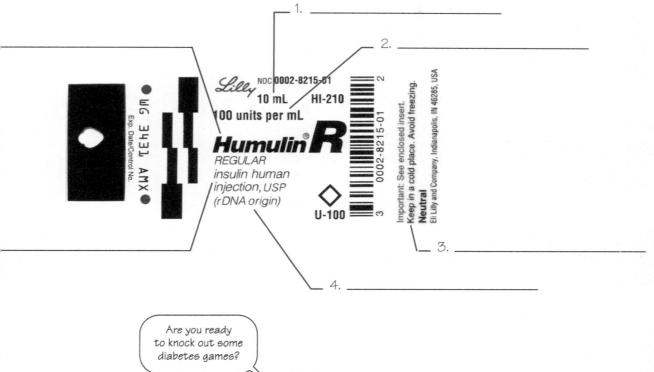

1. _____

2. _____

3. _____

4. _____

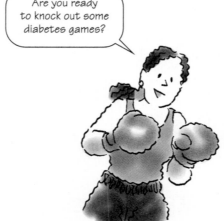

Are you ready to knock out some diabetes games?

Strikeout

Strike out the incorrect statements.

Diabetes is classified as type 1 or type 2.

Type 1 diabetes is also known as *non-insulin-dependent diabetes.*

Type 1 diabetes is typically diagnosed after age 30.

In type 2 diabetes, the pancreas produces some insulin, but it's too little or ineffective.

The incidence of Type 2 diabetes among children is declining.

Hit or miss

Label each statement with a "T" for "True" or an "F" for "False."

_____ 1. The anticoagulant heparin is used in large doses to prevent thrombosis and embolism.

_____ 2. The anticoagulant heparin is used in large doses to treat thrombosis and embolism.

_____ 3. Dosage calculation errors with heparin can cause excessive bleeding.

_____ 4. Heparin is available in one concentration.

Batter's box

Fill in the blanks with the correct answer options regarding insulin.

Insulin is classified according to its origin (human or _____) and action
1

time. Some insulins are derived from _____ pancreas and differ from
2

human insulin by _____ amino acids. Others are identical to human
3

insulin and are produced by _____ conversion of pork insulin or by
4

_____ deoxyribonucleic acid techniques. The origin appears on the
5

_____ label. Most insulin labels also contain an initial after the
6

_____ name, indicating the type of insulin. These different types of
7

insulin vary in onset, _____ , and duration of action. The initial R is for
8

_____ insulin; L is for _____ insulin; U is for
9 10

_____ insulin; and NPH is for neutral protamine Hagedorn.
11

Options

A. lente

B. animal

C. enzymatic

D. pork

E. peak

F. regular

G. trade

H. drug

I. recombinant

J. ultralente

K. two

Strikeout

Strike out the incorrect statements.

Insulin preparations are modified by combination with larger, insoluble protein molecules to slow absorption and prolong activity.

Insulin doses are expressed in units.

Insulin doses are available in three concentrations.

U-100 insulin is the most common concentration.

U-500 insulin is called *universal*.

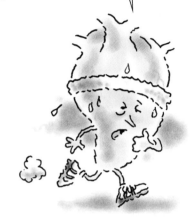

Do you think some insulin might help regulate my glucose levels after this workout?

Match point

Match the insulin syringe in Column 1 with its corresponding description in Column 2.

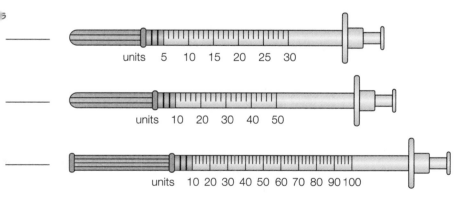

units 5 10 15 20 25 30

units 10 20 30 40 50

units 10 20 30 40 50 60 70 80 90 100

Options

A. The only type of insulin syringe available in the United States.

B. ³⁄₁₀-ml syringe

C. ½-ml syringe

Pep talk

"If I have ever made any valuable discoveries, it has been owing more to patient attention than to any other talent.

—Isaac Newton

Hit or miss

Label each statement with a "T" for "True" or an "F" for "False."

_____ 1. Regular insulin's onset is ½ hour, peak is 2 to 4 hours, and duration is 6 to 8 hours.

_____ 2. Lispro insulin peaks in ½ to 1½ hours.

_____ 3. Insulin zinc suspension (lente) is considered rapid acting.

_____ 4. Isophane insulin suspension (NPH) has an onset of ½ hour.

_____ 5. Regular insulin is considered intermediate acting.

_____ 6. Isophane 70%, regular insulin 30% peaks in 2 to 12 hours.

_____ 7. Isophane 50%, regular insulin 50% has a duration of 24 hours.

_____ 8. Extended insulin zinc suspension (ultralente) peaks in 4 to 8 hours.

_____ 9. Insulin glargine (Lantus) has an onset of 1 hour.

_____ 10. Lantus is considered long acting.

Batter's box

Fill in the blanks with the correct answer options regarding insulin orders.

For a newly diagnosed, ill, or _____ diabetic patient, the
                                        1

practitioner may write an order for insulin on a _____
                                                        2

scale. This type of order individualizes the insulin

_____ and administration times according to the pa-
        3

tient's _____ , activity level, work habits, desired degree
            4

of blood glucose control, and _____ to insulin prepara-
                                        5

tions.

Options
A. sliding
B. response
C. doses
D. age
E. unstable

Order up!
Insulin orders
should be
read over
carefully.

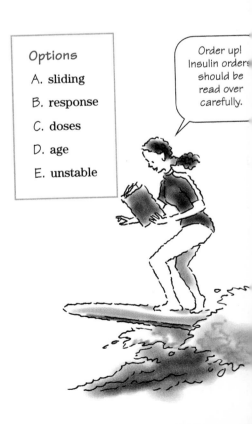

Starting lineup

The practitioner has ordered regular insulin mixed with NPH insulin to be injected together at the same site. Put the steps for drawing up the insulin into the right order.

Recheck the drug order.

Roll the NPH vial between your palms to mix it thoroughly.

Read the vial labels carefully.

Clean the tops of both vials of insulin with alcohol swabs.

Inject into the regular insulin vial an amount of air equal to the dose of the regular insulin. Then withdraw the prescribed amount of regular insulin into the syringe.

Mix the insulins in the syringe.

Inject air into the NPH vial equal to the amount of insulin you need to give. Withdraw the needle and syringe, but don't withdraw any NPH insulin.

Clean the top of the NPH vial again. Then insert the needle of the syringe containing the regular insulin into the vial, and withdraw the prescribed amount of NPH insulin.

Match point

The practitioner orders 8,500 units of heparin subQ q12h. The heparin you have available contains 10,000 units/ml. Match the steps Column 1 with their corresponding equation steps in Column 2 to figure out how many milliliters of heparin you should give.

Clues

1. Step 1 _____
2. Step 2 _____
3. Step 3 _____
4. Step 4 _____
5. Step 5 _____

Options

A. Set up the second ratio with the desired dose and unknown amount of heparin.

B. Put the first and second ratios into a proportion.

C. Set up the first ratio with the known heparin concentration.

D. Solve for *X* by dividing each side of the equation by 10,000 units and canceling units that appear in both the numerator and denominator.

E. Set up an equation by multiplying the means and extremes.

Aim for no errors when you're following orders for insulin and unit-based drugs.

Finish line

Use this insulin sliding scale to fill in the correct answers below.

Blood glucose level	Insulin dose
< 200 mg/dl	No insulin
201 to 250 mg/dl	2 units regular insulin
251 to 300 mg/dl	4 units regular insulin
301 to 350 mg/dl	6 units regular insulin
351 to 400 mg/dl	8 units regular insulin
> 400 mg/dl	Call doctor for insulin order.

1. If the patient's blood glucose level is 180 mg/dl, then his insulin dose should be _____ .
2. If the patient's blood glucose level is 224 mg/dl, then his insulin dose should be _____ .
3. If the patient's blood glucose level is 256 mg/dl, then his insulin dose should be _____ .
4. If the patient's blood glucose level is 345 mg/dl, then his insulin dose should be _____ .
5. If the patient's blood glucose level is 376 mg/dl, then his insulin dose should be _____ .
6. If the patient's blood glucose level is 450 mg/dl, then his insulin dose should be _____ .

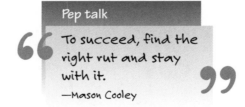

Pep talk

To succeed, find the right rut and stay with it.
—Mason Cooley

■■
■ Batter's box

Fill in the blanks with the correct answer options regarding reconstituting powders.

Some drugs are manufactured and packaged as powders because they become unstable

quickly when they're in _____ . When the practitioner prescribes such a

1

drug, either you or the pharmacist must _____ it before it can be admin-

2

istered. Powders come in single-strength or multiple-strength _____ .

3

A single-strength powder—such as levothyroxine sodium—may be reconstituted to

only one dose strength per _____ route, as specified by the manufacturer.

4

A multiple-strength powder—such as _____—can be reconstituted to

5

_____ dose strengths by adjusting the amounts of diluent.

6

When reconstituting a multiple-strength powder, check the _____ label

7

or package insert for the dose-strength _____ and choose the one that's

8

_____ to the ordered dose strength.

9

Options
A. closest
B. drug
C. formulations
D. administration
E. various
F. reconstitute
G. options
H. penicillin
I. solution

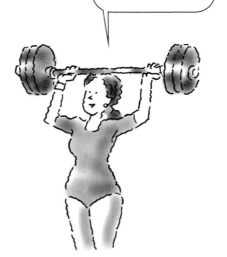

Reconstituted
drugs change from
one form to another.
I hope all this time in
the gym does the
same for me!

Finish line

Label each part of this two-chamber vial.

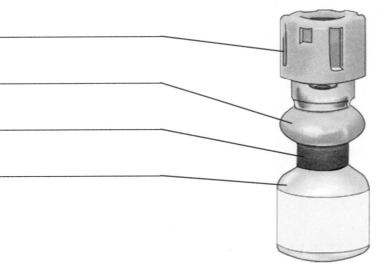

Mix up your reconstitution plays to make it to the end zone!

Strikeout

Strike out the incorrect statements.

When reconstituting a powder for injection, begin by checking the label of the powder container.

The label of the powder container tells you the quantity of drug in a vial or ampule, the amount and type of diluent to add to the powder, and the strength and expiration date of the resulting solution.

When a diluent is added to a powder, the fluid volume decreases.

The label of the powder container calls for more diluent than the total volume of prepared solution.

■ Hit or miss

Label each statement with a "T" for "True" or an "F" for "False."

_____ 1. Some drugs that need reconstitution are packaged in vials with two chambers separated by a plunger.

_____ 2. The upper chamber of the two-chamber vial contains the diluent, and the lower chamber contains the powdered drug.

_____ 3. When the top of the vial is depressed, the stopper dislodges, allowing the diluent to flow into the upper chamber, where it can be mixed with the powdered drug.

_____ 4. After you depress the top of the vial, and dislodge the chamber, you can remove the correct amount of solution with a syringe.

_____ 5. To determine how much solution to give, refer to the drug label for information about the dose strength of a prepared solution.

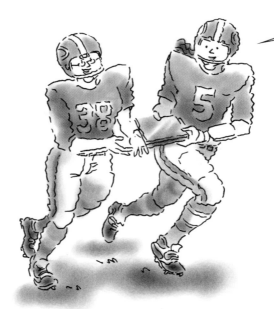

Keep scoring big points with your knowledge of reconstitution!

■ Strikeout

Strike out the incorrect statements.

1. If the information about a drug dose's strength isn't on the label, you should check the package insert.

2. The package inserts that are included with drugs don't usually provide information other than what is on the outer label.

3. The package insert or label of a drug will also list the type of diluent needed.

4. The package insert or label of a drug will also list the dose strength after reconstitution.

5. The package insert or label of a drug will also list special instructions about administration.

Hit or miss

Label each statement with a "T" for "True" or an "F" for "False."

_ 1. When you reconstitute a powder that comes in multiple strengths, you should be especially careful in choosing the most appropriate strength for the prescribed dose.

_ 2. After you've reconstituted a drug, it isn't necessary to label it.

_ 3. After you've reconstituted a drug, you should label it with your initials and the reconstitution date.

_ 4. After you've reconstituted a drug, you should label it with the expiration date and the dose strength only.

Starting lineup

The practitioner prescribes 300 mg chlorothiazide for your patient but the only available vial holds 500 mg. The drug label says to add 18 ml of sterile water to yield 500 mg/20 ml. Put the equation steps in the correct order to figure out how much solution you should administer after reconstitution.

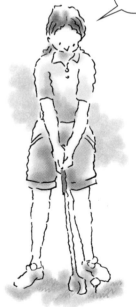

Practicing your equations will get you a hole in one every time.

$$\dfrac{300 \text{ mg}}{X}$$

$$\dfrac{500 \text{ mg}}{20 \text{ ml}}$$

$$\dfrac{0 \text{ ml} \times 300 \text{ mg}}{500 \text{ mg}} = \dfrac{X \times 500 \text{ mg}}{500 \text{ mg}}$$

$$X = \dfrac{6000 \text{ ml}}{500}$$

$$X = 12 \text{ ml}$$

$$\dfrac{500 \text{ mg}}{20 \text{ ml}} = \dfrac{300 \text{ mg}}{X}$$

$$0 \text{ ml} \times 300 \text{ mg} = X \times 500 \text{ mg}$$

■■
■ Match point

The practitioner orders 1 g ceftriaxone for your patient. A 2-g vial of powdered ceftriaxone is available. The label says to add 19.2 ml sterile water to yield 100mg/1ml. Match the steps Column 1 with its corresponding equation step in Column 2 to figure out how many milliliters of reconstituted ceftriaxone you should give.

Clues

1. Step 1 _____

2. Step 2 _____

3. Step 3 _____

4. Step 4 _____

5. Step 5 _____

Options

A. Set up the second fraction with the desired dose and the unknown amount of solution.

B. Set up the first fraction with the known ceftriaxone concentration.

C. Solve for *X* by dividing each side of the equation by 2,000 mg and canceling units that appear in both the numerator and denominator.

D. Put the first and second fractions into a proportion, making sure the same units of measures appear in both numerators.

E. Cross-multiply the fractions.

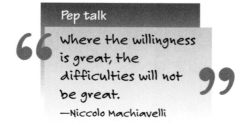

Pep talk

“Where the willingness is great, the difficulties will not be great.

—Niccolo Machiavelli

6

Calculating I.V. infusions

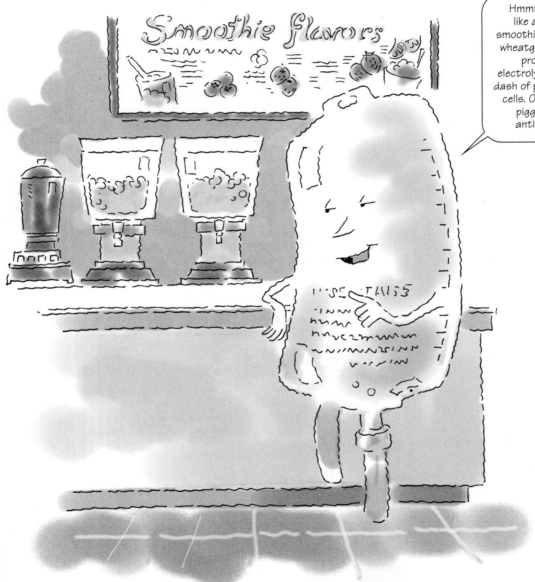

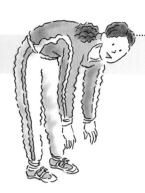

■ Warm-up

Calculating I.V. infusions review

Drip rate

- Represents the number of drops infused per minute
- Formula to use: Total milliliters ÷ total minutes × drop factor in drops (gtt)/milliliter
- Drop factor represents the number of drops per milliliters of solution that the I.V. tubing is designed to deliver

Flow rate

- Represents the number of milliliters of fluid administered over 1 hour
- Formula to use: Total volume ordered ÷ number of hours

Drip rate shortcut

Macrodrips

- For 10 gtt/ml sets, divide hourly flow rate by 6
- For 15 gtt/ml sets, divide hourly flow rate by 4
- For 20 gtt/ml sets, divide hourly flow rate by 3

Microdrips

- Drip rate = flow rate

Infusion time

- The amount of time required for infusion of a specified volume of I.V. fluid
- Method #1: infusion time = infusion volume ÷ flow rate
- Method #2: infusion time = infused volume ÷ drip rate/drop factor × 60 minutes

Regulating I.V. flow manually

- Count the number of drops going into the drip chamber.
- Adjust the flow with the roller clamp to the appropriate drip rate.
- Time-tape the I.V. bag.

Regulating I.V. flow with electronic infusion pumps

- Program the device based on the infusion rate.
- Count drips in the chamber to check the infusion.

PCA pump

- Allows the patient to self-administer an analgesic
- Also can be programmed to deliver a basal dose of drug

- Requires use of an access code or key to prevent unauth rized use of the device

Using a PCA pump

- Draw drug into a syringe and insert into the PCA pump.
- Program the pump according to manufacturer's direction
- Read the PCA log; then record information per facility p cy.

PCA log notes

- Strength of drug solution in syringe
- Number of drug administrations during assessment peri
- Basal dose patient received, if any
- Amount of solution received (equals the number of injec tions × volume of injections + basal doses)
- Total amount of drug received (equals total amount of so tion × solution strength)

Heparin flow rate formula

- First determine the solution's concentration: Divide unit drug added by the amount of solution in milliliters.
- Then state as a fraction (the desired dose over the unkno flow rate).
- Lastly, cross-multiply and solve for X.

Insulin infusions

- Regular insulin is the only type administered by I.V. rout
- Use an infusion pump.
- Use concentrations of 1 unit/ml.

Electrolyte and nutrient infusions

- Make sure that drugs to be infused together are compati
- Calculate the amount of additive using the proportion method as you would for any prepared liquid drug.
- Calculate the flow rate and the drip rate.

Blood infusions

- Filter out agglutinated cells with special administration s
- Drop factor is 10 to 15 gtt/ml.
- Use at least an 18G I.V. catheter.

TPN administration

- Can be given centrally or peripherally
- Initially infused at 40 ml/hour, then increased to maintenance
- Administered with an infusion pump

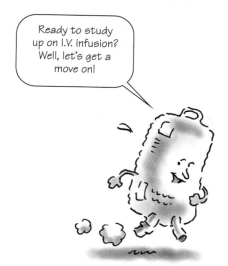

Ready to study up on I.V. infusion? Well, let's get a move on!

Batter's box

Fill in the blanks with the correct answer options regarding I.V. infusions.

Careful administration of _____ fluids is critical, especially when

dealing with patients who are susceptible to _____ volume changes.

_____ infusion of I.V. fluids or blood products may seriously threaten
3

your patient's health. To administer I.V. fluids safely, you need information specifying

how much fluid to give, the correct length of time for _____ , the type
4

of fluid, and what may be _____ to the fluid. Start by examining the
5

outside of a full I.V. bag and learn to identify all of its _____ .
6

Next, you'll need to be able to select the proper _____ , calculate drip
7

rates and _____ rates, and become comfortable working with I.V.
8

equipment such as _____ infusion devices.
9

Options

A. administration

B. components

C. I.V.

D. electronic

E. rapid

F. tubing

G. flow

H. fluid

I. added

▪️ Finish line

Label each part of the outside of the I.V. bag.

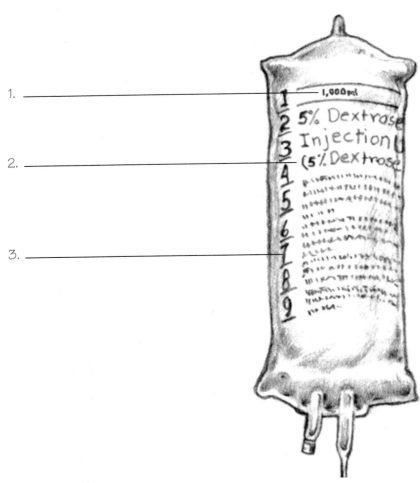

1. _____

2. _____

3. _____

Batter's box

Fill in the blanks with the correct answer options regarding I.V. tubing selection.

ecting I.V. tubing plays an important role in _____ I.V.
<u>1</u>

sion rates. Most facilities stock I.V. tubing in _____
<u>2</u>

es: microdrip and _____ . Microdrip tubing, as its name
<u>3</u>

lies, delivers _____ drops than macrodrip. Microdrip
<u>4</u>

delivers _____ drops per minute.
<u>5</u>

> Options
>
> A. macrodrip
>
> B. smaller
>
> C. two
>
> D. more
>
> E. calculating

> Whether you're in or out of water, selecting the right tube is pretty important!

Hit or miss

Label each statement with a "T" for "True" or an "F" for "False."

___ 1. If the infusion rate for a solution is relatively fast, you should select macrodrip tubing.

___ 2. If the infusion rate for a solution is 40 ml/hour, you should select macrodrip tubing.

___ 3. If you use macrodrip tubing for a slow infusion, maintaining accurate flow may be difficult, if not impossible.

■■
■ Strikeout

Cross out the incorrect statement.

1. You should use macrodrip tubing for infusions of at least 80 ml/hour.
2. You should use macrodrip tubing for infusions for pediatric patients.
3. With electronic infusion devices, you should select the tubing specifically made to work with those devices.

■■
■ Match point

Match the terms in Column 1 with their corresponding descriptions in Column 2.

Clues

1. Drip rate _____
2. Calibration _____
3. Drop factor _____
4. Standard (macrodrip) administration _____
5. Standard microdrip (minidrip) set _____

Options

A. The number of drops per milliliter of solution calibrated for an administration set
B. The number of drops of solution to infuse per minute
C. The drop factor is 60 gtt/ml
D. Something you need to know to calculate the drip rate
E. The drop factor is usually 10, 15, or 20 gtt/ml

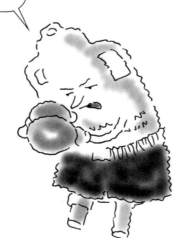

Knock everyone out with your ability to calculate drip rates!

Batter's box

Fill in the blanks with the correct information regarding one formula for calculating drip rates.

Drip rate in _____ /minute =
₁

total _____ /total _____ ×
₂   ₃

drop _____ in drops/ml.
₄

Options

A. factor

B. drops

C. milliliters

D. minutes

Now stretch your abilities with a drip rate calculation problem.

Starting lineup

Your patient needs an infusion of normal saline solution at 175 ml/hour. If the tubing set is calibrated at 15 gtt/ml, list the steps below in the order that you would need to calculate the drip rate.

$$X = \frac{175 \text{ ml}}{60 \text{ minutes}} \times \frac{15 \text{ gtt}}{\text{ml}}$$

$$X = \frac{175 \times 15\text{gtt}}{60 \text{ minutes}}$$

$$X = \frac{2{,}625 \text{ gtt}}{60 \text{ minutes}}$$

$$X = \frac{43.75 \text{ gtt}}{\text{minute}}$$

$$\frac{175 \text{ ml}}{60 \text{ minutes}}$$

Convert 1 hour to 60 minutes to fit the formula.

Pep talk

" Just don't give up trying to do what you really want to do. Where there is love and inspiration, I don't think you can go wrong.

—Ella Fitzgerald "

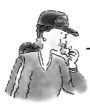

Coaching session
Checking an I.V.

Save time by assessing your patient's I.V. infusion at the beginning of every shift.
• Are the time, volume, and rate labeled correctly? If so, do they match the order?
• Check maintenance fluids and drug infusions, such as insulin, dopamine, and morphine. Are the additives correct? Are they in the right solutions?

• After calculating the drug dosage, check the bag again to verify that the solution is labeled with the time, name, and amount of drug added.
• If an electronic infusion device is being used, is it set correctly?
• Examine the tubing from the bag down to the patient to see whether the drug is infusing into the correct I.V. port. This is critical when a patient had multiple lines.

■ Batter's box

Fill in the blanks with the correct information regarding calculating the drip rate for an order that reads: *magnesium sulfate 2 gm in 100 ml NS over 60 minutes, using an infusion pump for the infusion, along with a tubing set calibrated at 60 gtt/ml*

Set up the fraction. Place the _____ of the infusion in the
                                              1

numerator. Place the number of _____ for the infusion in
                                              2

the denominator. To determine the number of _____ per
                                                         3

minute to be infused (solve for *X*), multiply the _____ by
                                                              4

the drop factor. Cancel units that appear in both the numerator and

denominator. To solve for _____ , divide the
                                    5

_____ by the _____ . The drip rate is
        6   7

100 gtt/minute.

> Options
>
> A. drops
> B. *X*
> C. volume
> D. denominator
> E. minutes
> F. numerator
> G. fraction

Let's keep these calculations running smoothly!

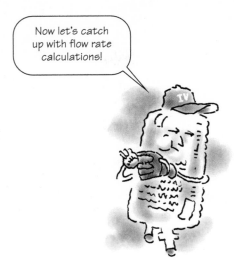

Hit or miss

Label each statement with a "T" for "True" or an "F" for "False."

___ 1. If your patient is receiving a large-volume infusion to maintain hydration or to replace fluids or electrolytes, it's possible that you may need to calculate the flow rate.

___ 2. The flow rate is the number of milliliters of fluid to administer over 2 hours.

___ 3. The flow rate may also refer to the number of milliliters of fluid to administer per minute.

___ 4. To calculate the flow rate, you need to know the total volume to be infused in milliliters and the amount of time for the infusion.

___ 5. To calculate the flow rate, use the formula of numbers of hours/total volume ordered.

Batter's box

Fill in the blanks with the correct information regarding performing the calculation.

ır patient needs 750 ml of fluid over 6 hours. Find the flow rate by

_____ the volume by the number of _____ .
   1   2

w rate = _____ ml/ _____ hours =
             3   4

_____ ml/hour.
   5

Options
A. 6
B. 750
C. dividing
D. hours
E. 125

Match point

Match the first half of each rule for calculating drip rates in Column 1 with its corresponding second half in Column 2.

Clues

1. For macrodrip sets that deliver 10 gtt/ml, _____
2. For macrodrip sets that deliver 15 gtt/ml, _____
3. For macrodrip sets that deliver 20 gtt/ml, _____
4. With a microdrip set with a drop factor of 60 gtt/ml, _____

Options

A. divide the hourly flow rate by 4.
B. divide the hourly flow rate by 6.
C. the drip rate is the same as the flow ra
D. divide the hourly flow rate by 3.

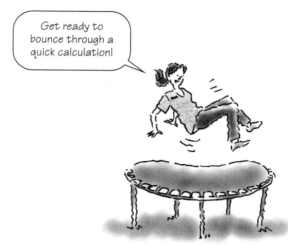

Hit or miss

Label the statement with a "T" for "True" or an "F" for "False."

Statement: Your patient needs 500 ml of normal saline solution over 4 hours. The flow rate is 125 ml/hour.

Answer: _____

Pep talk

" What we hope ever to
do with ease, we
must learn first to
do with diligence. "
—Samuel Johnson

Batter's box

Fill in the blanks with the correct information regarding the equation.

For a solution with a flow rate of 125 ml/hour (125 ml/ _____ minutes)
                                                          1

when using a _____ set (drop factor of 60 gtt/ml), note that the number
              2

of minutes and the number of _____ per milliliter cancel each other
                               3

out. The drip rate (_____ gtt/minute) is the same as the number of
                      4

milliliters of fluid per hour (_____ rate).
                                 5

> We'd say this flow rate is pretty high!

Options

A. 125

B. 60

C. microdrip

D. flow

E. drops

Starting lineup

The practitioner prescribes 750 ml of normal saline to be infused over 8 hours. If your administration set delivers 15 gtt/ml, list the steps below in the order that you would need to calculate the drip rate.

Remember the rule: for a set that delivers 15 gtt/ml, divide the flow rate by 4 to determine the drip rate.	
Determine the flow rate (X) by dividing the number of milliliters to be delivered by the number of hours.	
Set up an equation to determine the drip rate, which now becomes X, and solve for X. Divide the flow rate by 4.	

■■
■ Strikeout

Cross out the incorrect statement.

1. After calculating the drip and flow rate, it's possible to compute the time required for infusion of a specified volume of I.V. fluid.

2. Computing the time required for infusion of a specified volume of I.V. fluid helps keep the infusion on schedule.

3. Computing the time required for infusion of a specified volume of I.V. fluid won't help you perform laboratory tests on time.

4. To calculate the infusion time, you must know the flow rate in milliliters per hour and the volume to be infused.

5. The formula to calculate infusion rate is infusion time = flow rate/volume to be infused.

■■
■ Batter's box

Fill in the blanks with the correct information regarding calculating infusion time.

Your patient is to receive an I.V. infusion of 150 ml/hour using a 60 gtt/ml set.

To calculate the drip rate, determine the _____ rate first. The
                                              1

flow rate is the number of _____ of fluid to administer over
                                  2

_____ hour, so it's _____ ml/hour. Remember
         3   4

that with a microdrip set, the drip rate is the _____ as the flow
                                                        5

rate. Thus, the drip rate is 150 gtt/ _____ .
                                           6

Options
A. flow
B. milliliters
C. minute
D. 150
E. 1
F. same

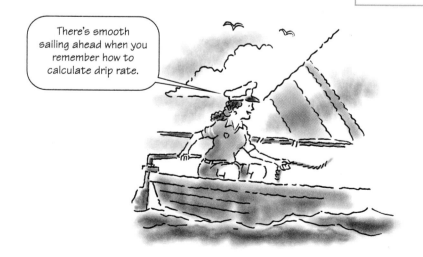

There's smooth sailing ahead when you remember how to calculate drip rate.

Starting lineup

If you plan to infuse 500 ml of normal saline solution at 50 ml/hour, list the steps below in the order that you would need to calculate the infusion time.

Set up the fraction with the volume of the infusion as the numerator and the flow rate as the denominator.	
Solve for X by dividing 500 by 50 and canceling units that appear in both the numerator and denominator.	

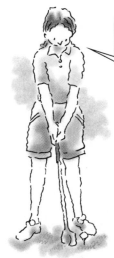

Having to brush up on infusion rate calculation really tees me off, but a little practice will do me good.

Dosage drills

Test your math skills with this drill.

Be sure to show how you arrive at your answer.

A fluid challenge is ordered for a patient in hypovolemic shock. He needs 500 ml of normal saline solution over 2 hours. What should the nurse set the infusion rate at?

Your answer: _____

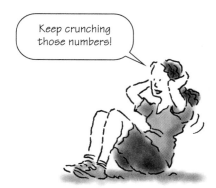

■ Hit or miss

Label the statement with a "T" for "True" or an "F" for "False."

Statement: Your patient requires 450 ml of normal saline at 90 ml/hour. If the normal saline solution is hung at 5 a.m.
the infusion will be completed at 1:15 a.m.

Answer: _____

■ Batter's box

Fill in the blanks with the correct components of this infusion formula.

Suppose all you know about a particular I.V. fluid are the volume to
be infused, the drip rate, and the drop factor. You would then use
the following alternative formula to calculate the infusion time:

Infusion time in _____ = _____ to be
                        1   2

infused/(_____ rate/ _____ factor) ×
                3   4

60 _____
         5

> **Options**
> A. volume
> B. hours
> C. drop
> D. drip
> E. minutes

Pep talk

> The ability to think straight, some
> knowledge of the past, some vision
> of the future, some urge to fit
> that service into the well-being
> of the community—these are the
> most vital things education must
> try to produce.
> —Virginia Gildersleeve

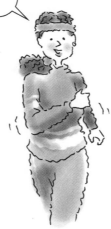

Keep up the pace with another set of equations!

Dosage drills

Test your math skills with this drill.

Be sure to show how you arrive at your answer.

At 6:00 a.m., a patient receives a preoperative infusion of 1,000 ml of dextrose 5% in half-normal saline solution at 125 ml/hr, followed by 1,000 ml of dextrose 5% in water at 100 ml/hr. What's the total infusion time?

Your answer: _____

Starting lineup

A practitioner prescribes 500 ml of normal saline I.V. at 64 gtt/minute. The drop factor is 15 gtt/ml. List the steps below in order that you would need to calculate the infusion time.

$$X = \dfrac{500 \, \cancel{ml}}{\dfrac{4.27 \, \cancel{ml}}{1 \, \cancel{min}} \times \dfrac{60 \, \cancel{min}}{1 \, hour}}$$

$$X = \dfrac{500}{4.27 \times 60 \, hours}$$

$$X = \dfrac{500}{256.2 \, hours}$$

$$\text{Infusion time} = \dfrac{500 \, ml}{\left(\dfrac{64 \, gtt/minute}{15 \, gtt/minute}\right) \times 60 \, minutes}$$

$$X = \dfrac{500}{256 \, hours}$$

$$X = 1.95 \, hours$$

$$\dfrac{64 \, \cancel{gtt}}{1 \, min} \times \dfrac{1 \, ml}{15 \, \cancel{gtt}} = \dfrac{64 \, ml}{15 \, min} = 4.27 \, ml/min$$

$$1.95 \, hours \times 60 \, minutes = 117 \, minutes$$

$$X = 1 \, hour \, 57 \, minutes$$

Hit or miss

Label the statement with a "T" for "True" or an "F" for "False."

Statement: If 250 ml of hetastarch (Hespan) are infusing at 20 gtt/minute through tubing with a calibration of 10 gtt/ml, the infusion time is 4 hours and 10 minutes.

Answer: _____

> Now you're getting into the heavy lifting of equation work.

Dosage drills

Test your math skills with this drill.

> Be sure to show how you arrive at your answer.

One liter of dextrose 5% in half-normal saline solution was hung at 1000, infusing at 100 ml/hr. It's now 1400. How much fluid should remain in the I.V. bag?

Your answer: _____

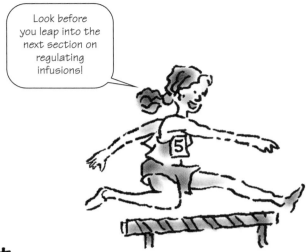

Look before you leap into the next section on regulating infusions!

■ Strikeout

Cross out the incorrect statements.

1. You can only regulate I.V. flow by using a pump.
2. You can only regulate I.V. flow manually.
3. You can use a patient-controlled analgesia pump to regulate I.V. flow.
4. To manually regulate I.V. flow, you should count the number of drops going into the drip chamber.
5. While counting the drops that go into the drip chamber, you should adjust the flow with the roller clamp until the fluid is infusing at the appropriate number of drops per minute.

■ Batter's box

Fill in the blanks with the correct information regarding manual regulation of I.V. flow.

When counting drops while manually regulating I.V. flow, don't count for a

_____ minute—calculate the drip rate for _____ seconds
       1   2

only. To do this, _____ the prescribed drip rate by _____
                 3   4

(because 15 seconds is ¼ of a minute). Afterward, _____ the I.V. bag
                                                          5

to ensure that the solution is given at the prescribed rate and to make recording fluid

intake easier.

Options

A. full

B. divide

C. time-tape

D. 15

E. 4

Batter's box

Fill in the blanks with the correct information regarding electronic infusion pumps.

tronic infusion pumps _____ I.V. administration. Pumps administer fluid
                               1

er _____ pressure and are calibrated by _____ rate and
          2   3

me. When using a pump, set the device to deliver a _____ amount of
                                                              4

tion per hour, following the manufacturer's directions. Electronic infusion pumps offer

y advantages, such as:

owing you easy control of the rate, or _____ , by setting it on the machine
                                                  5

ortening the time needed to _____ an infusion rate
                                      6

quiring less maintenance than standard devices that drip fluid by _____
                                                                            7

oviding greater accuracy than _____ devices.
                                        8

Options
A. positive
B. calculate
C. standard
D. drip
E. volume
F. constant
G. facilitate
H. gravity

Now go train a little on the bag— the I.V. bag!

Hit or miss

Label each statement with a "T" for "True" or an "F" for "False."

_ 1. To time-tape an I.V. bag, you should place a strip of adhesive tape from the bottom to the top of the bag.

_ 2. When time-taping an I.V. bag, you should record the time that you hung the bag next to the "0" marking.

_ 3. When time-taping an I.V. bag, you should mark the time at which the solution will be completely infused at the top of the tape.

_ 4. You shouldn't write directly on the I.V. bag with a felt-tip marker because the ink may seep into the fluid.

_ 5. Some manufacturers provide printed time-tapes for use with their solutions.

■■ ■ Strikeout

Cross out the incorrect statements.

1. Most electronic infusion pumps keep track of the amount of fluid that has been infused.

2. Most electronic infusion pumps have alarms.

3. Currently there are no electronic infusion pumps that have devices which prevent them from pumping fluids into infiltrated sites.

4. When using an electronic pump to regulate I.V. flow, you should program the device based on your calculation of the infusion rate.

5. Electronic infusion pumps are foolproof.

6. You should check the infusion on an electronic infusion pump by counting the drips in the chamber.

■■ ■ Batter's box

Fill in the blanks with the correct information regarding electronic infusion pumps.

To determine the electronic infusion pump settings, consider the _____
1

of fluid to be given and the total _____ time. With most devices, you'll
2

need to _____ both the amount of _____ to be infused and
3   4

the _____ flow rate. However, some devices require you to program the
5

flow rate per _____ or the drip rate.
6

Options
A. infusion
B. volume
C. program
D. minute
E. hourly
F. fluid

I want to pump YOU up! In an electric infusion kind of way, of course.

Hit or miss

Label each statement with a "T" for "True" or an "F" for "False."

_ 1. The computerized PCA pump allows a patient to self-administer an analgesic by pushing a button.

_ 2. The patient programs the PCA pump to deliver a precise dose every time.

_ 3. The PCA pump can also be programmed to deliver a basal dose drug in addition to the patient-controlled dose.

_ 4. A disadvantage of using a PCA pump over the traditional approach is that blood concentrations of analgesics can be inconsistent throughout the day.

_ 5. With PCA pumps, patients tend to use less medication than they do with the traditional approach.

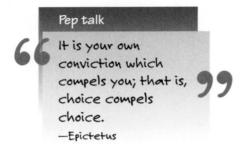

Pep talk

" It is your own conviction which compels you; that is, choice compels choice. "

—Epictetus

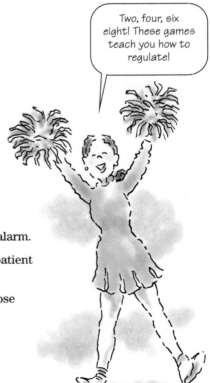

Two, four, six eight! These games teach you how to regulate!

Strikeout

Cross out the incorrect statements.

PCA pumps have several built-in safety features.

Drug dose is programmed on PCA pumps, but administration frequency is not.

If the patient tries to overmedicate himself, the PCA pump machine sounds an alarm.

Some PCA pumps record the number of requests and the number of times the patient actually receives medication.

PCA machines require you to use an access code or key before entering drug dose and frequency information into the system.

Some PCA machines record unauthorized entries.

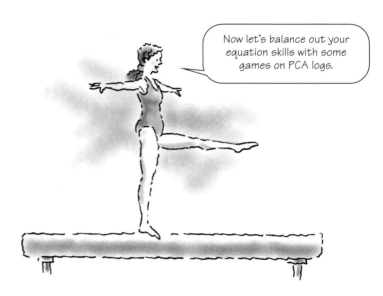

Now let's balance out your equation skills with some games on PCA logs.

Starting lineup

List the steps below in the order that you would need to follow when preparing a PCA pump for a patient.

Program the pump according to the manufacturer's directions.	
Draw the correct amount and concentration of the drug, and insert it into the PCA pump.	
Carefully read the PCA log, and then record the information based on your facility's policy.	

Hit or miss

Label each statement with a "T" for "True" or an "F" for "False."

_____ 1. When interpreting the PCA log, you should note the strength of the drug solution in the syringe.

_____ 2. You don't need to note the number of times the patient received the I.V. drug throughout the time covered by your assessment.

_____ 3. If your patient is receiving a basal dose, you should note that.

_____ 4. By multiplying the number of injections by the volume of the each injection and adding the basal dose, you can determine the amount of solution the patient received.

_____ 5. Fluid volume × solution strength = total medication received.

Strikeout

Cross out the incorrect statement.

Most facilities require the nurse who prepares the syringe to record the amount of fluid and drug in the syringe.

It isn't necessary for each nurse who checks the PCA log to double-check the amount of fluid and drug in the syringe.

The PCA record enables you to double-check the accuracy of everyone's calculations.

Batter's box

Fill in the blanks with the correct information regarding I.V. infusion rate.

I.V. infusion rate can change because the patient changed position, because the tubing became _____ , or because the drug _____

1
2

patient's skin. When problems occur you should recalculate the

_____ rate, taking into account the remaining _____

3
4

volume. If the fluid has infused too _____ , determine whether

5

patient can tolerate an increased rate by checking his cardiac and

_____ status. Look for a history of _____ insufficiency,

6
7

failure, _____ edema, or any other condition that increases the

8

of fluid overload. If the I.V. fluid has infused too _____ , slow or

9

the infusion and assess for signs of fluid overload, such as _____

10

increased blood pressure.

Options

A. infiltrated

B. kinked

C. quickly

D. slowly

E. crackles

F. renal

G. pulmonary

H. respiratory

I. time

J. drip

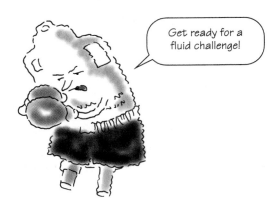

■ Match point

Match the information in Column 1 with its corresponding description in Column 2.

Clues

1. Fluid challenge _____
2. Fastest way to do a fluid challenge _____
3. Fluid bolus _____

Options

A. Used carefully in pediatric and elderly patients

B. The protocol for monitoring how a patient tolerates increased fluids

C. Involves increasing I.V. flow rate for a specified time and then reducing it to a maintenance rate

■ Hit or miss

Label each statement with a "T" for "True" or an "F" for "False."

_____ 1. The practitioner may prescribe heparin or insulin to be added to a large volume I.V. infusion.

_____ 2. Heparin or insulin may be ordered in milliliters per minute or units per minute.

_____ 3. To administer heparin or insulin safely, you must calculate the drug dose so that it falls within therapeutic limits.

_____ 4. Heparin hastens the formation of new clots and the development of pre-existing clots.

_____ 5. Each heparin dose is individualized based on the patient's coagulation status.

_____ 6. The patient's coagulation status when on heparin is measured by the partial thromboplastin time.

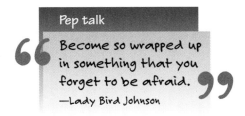

Pep talk

" Become so wrapped up in something that you forget to be afraid. "
—Lady Bird Johnson

Batter's box

Fill in the blanks with the correct information regarding flow rate.

urately calculating the flow rate of a heparin dose ensures that the dose falls within

e and _____ limits. This type of calculation _____ from
1   2

er flow rate calculations because it's used to administer a drug, not just a fluid. To

ulate the hourly heparin flow rate, first determine the solution's _____
3

_____ the _____ of drug added to the bag by the number
4   5

illiliters of solution. Then write a fraction stating the desired dose of heparin over

unknown _____ rate. Then simply cross-multiply to find the unknown
6

 rate.

Options
A. flow
B. concentration
C. dividing
D. differs
E. units
F. therapeutic

Dosage drills

Test your math skills with this drill.

Be sure to show
how you arrive at
your answer.

A patient with a myocardial infarction is receiving a lidocaine drip
containing 1 gram of lidocaine in 250 ml of dextrose 5% in water.
The drip factor is 15 gtt/ml. What should the nurse set the infusion
rate at in order to infuse 2 mg/min?

Your answer: _____

■■ ■ Starting lineup

An order states heparin 25,000 units in 1L of D$_5$W I.V. Infuse at 800 units/hr. List the steps below in the order that you wo
need to calculate the flow rate in milliliters per hour.

$$\frac{800 \text{ units/hour}}{X}$$

$$25,000 \text{ units} \times X = 800 \text{ units/hour} \times 1,000 \text{ ml}$$

$$\frac{25,000 \text{ units}}{1,000 \text{ ml}}$$

$$\frac{25,000 \text{ units} \times X}{25,000 \text{ units}} = \frac{800 \text{ units/hour} \times 1,000 \text{ ml}}{25,000 \text{ units}}$$

$$X = \frac{800,000 \text{ ml/hour}}{25,000}$$

$$X = 32 \text{ ml/hour}$$

$$\frac{25,000 \text{ units}}{1,000 \text{ ml}} = \frac{800 \text{ units/hour}}{X}$$

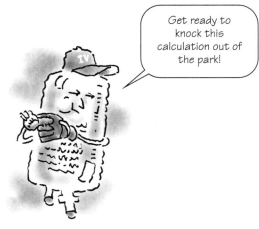

Get ready to
knock this
calculation out of
the park!

Dosage drills

Test your math skills with this drill.

Be sure to show
how you arrive at
your answer.

A practitioner's order reads "Give test dose of amphotericin B-
1 mg in 20 ml of dextrose 5% in water over 20 minutes."
How many milliliters per hour should the nurse set the
infusion pump to deliver?

Your answer: _____

Match point

You're about to administer a continuous infusion of 25,000 units of heparin in 250 ml or D$_5$W. If the patient is to receive 900 units/hour, what's the flow rate? To solve the equation, match the steps in Column 1 to the correct equation steps in Column 2.

Steps	Options
Step 1 _____	A. Put the first and second ratio into a proportion.
Step 2 _____	B. Write a ratio to express the known solution strength.
Step 3 _____	C. Write a ratio to describe the desired dose of heparin in relation to the unknown flow rate.
Step 4 _____	D. Solve for X by multiplying the extremes and the means.
Step 5 _____	E. Divide each side of the equation by 25,000 units and cancel units that appear in both the numerator and denominator.

■■
■ Starting lineup

A patient is receiving 10,000 units of heparin in 250 ml of D$_5$W I.V. The infusion rate is 30 ml/hour. List the steps below in the order that you would need to calculate the heparin dose he's receiving.

$$\frac{X}{30 \text{ ml/hour}}$$

$$X = 1{,}200 \text{ units/hour}$$

$$250 \text{ ml} \times X = 30 \text{ ml/hour} \times 10{,}000 \text{ units}$$

$$\frac{10{,}000 \text{ units}}{250 \text{ ml}}$$

$$\frac{\cancel{250 \text{ ml}} \times X}{\cancel{250 \text{ ml}}} = \frac{30 \text{ ml/hour} \times 10{,}000 \text{ units}}{250 \cancel{\text{ ml}}}$$

$$X = \frac{30 \times 10{,}000 \text{ units/hour}}{250}$$

$$\frac{10{,}000 \text{ units}}{250 \text{ ml}} = \frac{X}{30 \text{ ml/hour}}$$

$$X = \frac{300{,}000 \text{ units/hour}}{250}$$

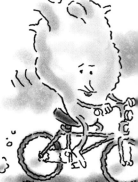

The more you try, the smoother the ride.

Hit or miss

Label each statement with a "T" for "True" or an "F" for "False."

___ 1. Continuous insulin infusion allows close control of insulin administration based on serial measurements of blood glucose levels.

___ 2. Nurses use infusion pumps to administer I.V. insulin.

___ 3. All types of insulin can be administered by the I.V. route.

___ 4. Insulin is usually prescribed in units per hour, but it may be ordered in milliliters per hour.

___ 5. An insulin I.V. infusion should be in a concentration of 5 units/ml.

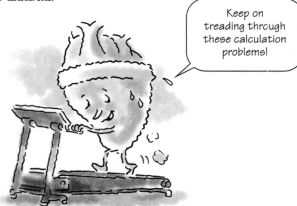

Keep on treading through these calculation problems!

Batter's box

Fill in the blanks with the correct equation options.

Question: Your patient needs a continuous infusion of 100 units of regular insulin in 100 ml of normal saline at 8 units/hour. What's the flow rate?

$$\frac{\boxed{} \text{ units}}{100 \text{ ml}}$$

$$\frac{8 \text{ units/hour}}{\boxed{}}$$

$$\frac{100 \text{ units}}{100 \; \boxed{}} = \frac{8 \text{ units/hour}}{X}$$

$$100 \text{ units} \times X = \frac{8 \; \boxed{}}{\text{hour}} \times 100 \text{ ml}$$

$$100 \text{ units} \times \frac{X}{100 \text{ units}} = \frac{8 \text{ units}}{\boxed{}} \times \frac{100 \text{ ml}}{100 \text{ units}}$$

$$X = \boxed{} \text{ ml/hour}$$

Options

A. 8

B. 100

C. hour

D. units

E. ml

F. X

■ Dosage drills

Test your math skills with this drill.

> Be sure to show how you arrive at your answer.

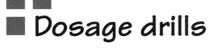

Normal saline solution is infusing at a rate of 62 gtt/min in a patient who has had a craniotomy for a brain tumor. The drip factor is 60 gtt/ml. How much fluid will infuse in 4 hours?

Your answer: _____

■ Starting lineup

Your patient is receiving a continuous infusion of 100 units of regular insulin in 100 ml of normal saline at 5 ml/hour. List the steps below in the order that you would need to calculate the number of units per hour your patient is receiving.

X : 5 ml/hour

X = 5 units/hour

100 units : 100 ml :: X : 5 ml/hour

100 units : 100 ml

$\dfrac{X \times \cancel{100\text{ml}}}{\cancel{100\text{ml}}} = \dfrac{\cancel{100}\text{ units} \times 5\,\cancel{\text{ml}}/\text{hour}}{\cancel{100\text{ml}}}$

$X \times 100\text{ ml}/100\text{ ml} = 100\text{ units} \times 5\text{ ml/hour}$

Hit or miss

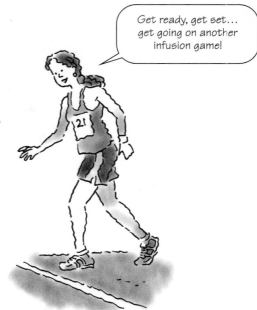

Get ready, get set... get going on another infusion game!

Label each statement with a "T" for "True" or an "F" for "False."

_ 1. Large-volume infusions with additives maintain or restore hydration or electrolyte status or supply additional electrolytes, vitamins or other nutrients.

_ 2. Potassium chloride, vitamins B and C, and trace elements are all examples of common additives.

_ 3. Electrolytes can be given in small-volume, intermittent doses administered I.M.

_ 4. It's never necessary to combine more than one additive in a solution.

_ 5. Before calculating the correct amount of each substance to inject into an electrolyte and nutrient infusion, you should check the compatibility chart or consult a pharmacist.

Strikeout

Cross out the incorrect statement.

If an additive isn't prepackaged in a solution, you must prepare the correct amount and add it to the solution.

If an additive isn't prepackaged in a solution, after preparing the correct amount and adding it to the solution, you must calculate the flow rate and the drip rate.

To calculate the amount of additive, use the fraction method.

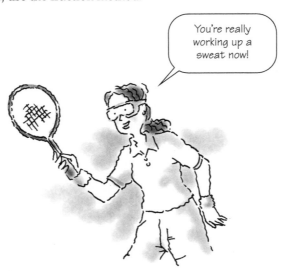

You're really working up a sweat now!

Starting lineup

Your patient requires 1,000 ml of D_5W with 75 mg of thiamine/L over 12 hours. The thiamine is available in a prepared syri of 50 mg/ml. List the steps below in the order that you would need to calculate how many milliliters of thiamine must be added to the solution and the flow rate.

75 mg : X

$X = 1.5$ ml

$X \times 50$ mg $= 75$ mg $\times 1$ ml

$\dfrac{X \times \cancel{50\ \text{mg}}}{\cancel{50\ \text{mg}}} = \dfrac{75\ \cancel{\text{mg}} \times 1\ \text{ml}}{50\ \cancel{\text{mg}}}$

50 mg : 1 ml :: 75 mg : X

50 mg : 1 ml

$\dfrac{1,000\ \text{ml}}{12\ \text{hr}} = 83.3$ ml/hr

$X = \dfrac{75\ \text{ml}}{50}$

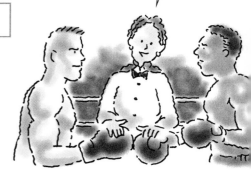

Punch your way through some piggyback infusions!

Batter's box

Fill in the blanks with the correct options regarding piggyback infusions.

An I.V. piggyback is a _____ -volume, intermittent infusion that's

         1

connected to an _____ I.V. line containing _____

       2   3

fluid. Most _____ contain antibiotics or _____ .

             4   5

To calculate piggyback infusions, use _____ .

                                 6

Options

A. existing

B. piggybacks

C. electrolytes

D. proportions

E. small

F. maintenance

Starting lineup

You receive an order for 250 mg of imipenem in 50 ml of normal saline solution to be infused over 1 hour. The imipenem vial contains 500 mg. The insert says to reconstitute the powder with 5 ml of normal saline solution. List the steps below in the order that you would need to calculate how much solution you should draw.

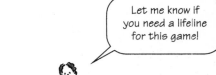

Let me know if you need a lifeline for this game!

$$X = \frac{250 \times 5 \text{ ml}}{500}$$

00 mg : 5 ml :: 250 mg : X

250 mg : X

$$\frac{\cancel{00 \text{ mg}} \times X}{\cancel{500 \text{ mg}}} = \frac{250 \cancel{\text{ mg}} \times 5 \text{ ml}}{\cancel{500 \text{ mg}}}$$

$$X = \frac{1{,}250 \text{ ml}}{500}$$

$X = 2.5$ ml

500 mg : 5 ml

0 mg $\times$ X = 250 mg $\times$ 5 ml

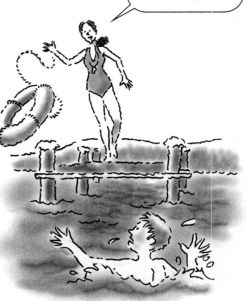

Hit or miss

Label the statement with a "T" for "True" or an "F" for "False."

tatement: You receive an order for 1000 mg of imipenem in 250 ml of normal saline solution to be infused over 1 hour. The imipenem vial contains 1,000 mg (1 g). The insert says to reconstitute the powder with 5 ml of normal saline solution. The flow rate is 250 ml/hour.

nswer: _____

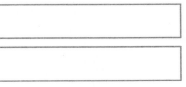

Pep talk

You may be disappointed if you fail, but you are doomed if you don't try.

—Beverly Sills

■■
■ Strikeout

Cross out the incorrect statement.

1. After calculating an I.V. piggyback dose, you should make sure that the drugs to be infused together are compatible.

2. After calculating an I.V. piggyback dose, it isn't necessary to make sure that the drugs mixed in the same syringe or I.V. bag are compatible.

3. If a drug compatibility chart isn't available for your use, you can substitute a drug handbook that includes a compatibility chart.

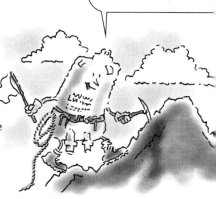

You're almost at the summit. Keep on going

■■
■ Dosage drills

Test your math skills with this drill.

Be sure to show how you arrive a your answer.

A practitioner orders 1 gram of vancomycin in 250 ml of dextrose 5% in water over 1 hour as endocarditis prophylaxis. What's the flow rate for this medication if the macrodrip administration set delivers 15 gtt/ml?

Your answer: _____

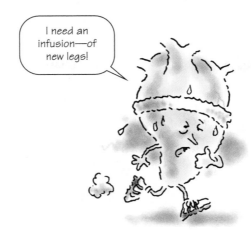

I need an infusion—of new legs!

Batter's box

Fill in the blanks with the correct options regarding blood and blood product infusions.

volume of fluid to be infused and the _____ factor can be used to calculate

$\underset{1}{}$

sfusions of blood and blood _____ . During such transfusions, take care to

$\underset{2}{}$

ent cell damage and ensure an adequate blood _____ by using a special

$\underset{3}{}$

inistration set that contains _____ to remove _____ cells.

$\underset{4}{} \qquad \underset{5}{}$

drop factor for these sets is usually 10 to 15 gtt/ml.

Options
A. agglutinated
B. filters
C. drop
D. products
E. flow

Hit or miss

Label each statement with a "T" for "True" or an "F" for "False."

__ 1. Generally, an 18G or larger I.V. catheter is used for administration of blood and blood products.

__ 2. The 18G or larger I.V. catheter can be used on all patients, regardless of age.

__ 3. A catheter smaller than 18G may be used for blood and blood product infusions on patients with chronic illnesses who are hospitalized frequently or severely dehydrated patients.

__ 4. A unit of whole blood or packed red blood cells should infuse for no longer than 6 hours.

■■ ■ Dosage drills

Test your math skills with this drill.

> Be sure to show how you arrive at your answer.

The order for a patient reads "250 ml hypertonic saline solution to run over 4 hours." What should the infusion rate be for this solution?

Your answer: _____

> Running over four hours?!? I think I'll sit this one out!

■■ ■ Batter's box

Fill in the blanks with the correct options regarding blood and blood product infusion precautions.

Take special precautions when transfusing blood products, such as

_____ , cryoprecipitate, and granulocytes. Consult your facility's
       1

procedure manual to find out the type of _____ to use and the
                                                2

rate and _____ of the transfusion. In addition, some medical
             3

conditions require the use of special tubing. For example, _____
                                                                    4

patients may need to use a _____ filter with blood products to
                                 5

prevent complications.

Options
A. tubing
B. duration
C. platelets
D. leukocyte
E. cancer

Starting lineup

Your patient is to receive 250 ml of packed red blood cells over 4 hours. The drop factor of the tubing is 10 gtt/ml. List the steps below in the order that you would need to calculate the drip rate in drops per minute.

Multiply the flow rate by the drop factor to find the drip rate in drops per minute.	
Find the flow rate in milliliters per minute.	

Batter's box

Fill in the blanks with the correct options regarding total parenteral nutrition.

_____ parenteral nutrition (TPN) refers to any nutrient
1

tion, including lipids, given through a _____ venous
2

TPN can be administered through a central vein, such as the

_____ vein or internal jugular vein. _____
3   4

nteral nutrition (PPN), which is administered through the veins of

_____ , legs, or scalp, supplies full caloric needs while
5

ding the risks that accompany a central line. Most facilities have a

ten protocol regarding _____ sites and recommended
6

tions for both TPN and PPN.

Options
A. arms
B. insertion
C. peripheral
D. total
E. central
F. subclavian

Coaching session
Total parenteral nutrition

- TPN is available as commercially prepared products or individually formulated solutions from the pharmacy. Solutions are prepared under sterile conditions to guard against patient infection. Very rarely are nurses responsible for preparing TPN solutions on the unit.
- TPN solutions contain a 10% or greater dextrose concentration. Amino acids are added to maintain or restore nitrogen bal-

ance, and vitamins, electrolytes, and trace minerals are added to meet individual patient needs.
- Lipids may also be added, but they're commonly given separately to prevent their destruction by the other nutrients. Remember that additives increase a solution's total volume, so they affect intake measurements.

Hit or miss

Label each statement with a "T" for "True" or an "F" for "False."

_____ 1. TPN is usually initially infused at 40 ml/hour.

_____ 2. After TPN is infused at a slow initial rate, it's rapidly increased to a maintenance level.

_____ 3. The rate of TPN infusion is gradually decreased before discontinuing TPN.

_____ 4. To set the maintenance flow rate of a TPN infusion pump, you must find the flow rate per minute.

_____ 5. To find the hourly flow rate on a TPN infusion, divide the amount to be infused daily by 24 hours.

Pep talk

The best things in life must come by effort from within, not by gifts from the outside.

—Fred Corson

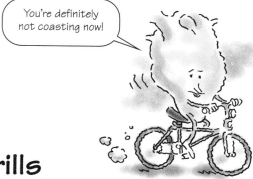

You're definitely not coasting now!

Dosage drills

Test your math skills with this drill.

Be sure to show how you arrive at your answer.

A practitioner's order reads Heparin I.V. at 1,400 units/hr. The pharmacy sends heparin in a bag containing 25,000 units in 250 ml of dextrose 5% in water. What infusion rate should be set on the I.V. pump?

Your answer: _____

Starting lineup

Your patient needs 22.5 ml of erythromycin, which is equal to 750 mg. The infusion is to be completed in 60 minutes using a tubing set calibrated to 20 gtt/ml. List the steps below in the order that you would need to calculate the drip rate.

$X = 7.5$ gtt/minute

$= \dfrac{22.5 \text{ ml}}{60 \text{ minutes}} \times 20 \text{ gtt/ml}$

$X = \dfrac{450 \text{ gtt}}{60 \text{ minute}}$

$\dfrac{22.5 \text{ ml}}{60 \text{ minutes}}$

$X = \dfrac{22.5 \times 20 \text{ gtt}}{60 \text{ minutes}}$

Dosage drills

Test your math skills with this drill.

Be sure to show how you arrive at your answer.

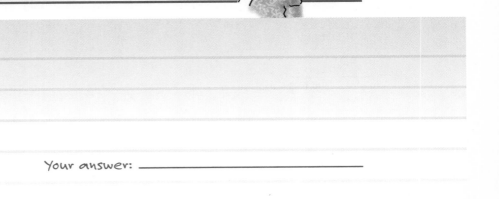

An I.V. of dextrose 5% in half-normal saline solution with 40 mEq potassium chloride is infusing at 40 ml/hr in a patient with Kaposi's sarcoma. How much fluid will the patient receive in 8 hours?

Your answer: _____

Dosage drills

Test your math skills with this drill.

> Be sure to show how you arrive at your answer.

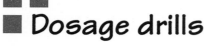

A patient with multiple myeloma is receiving 400 mg of morphine sulfate in 100 ml of normal saline solution at 2 ml/hr. How many milligrams per hour is the patient receiving?

Your answer: _____

Starting lineup

If you infuse 750 ml of lactated Ringer's solution at 50 gtt/minute using a set calibration of 10 gtt/ml, list the steps below in the order that you would need to calculate the infusion time.

$$\frac{50 \ \text{gtt}}{1 \ \text{min}} \times \frac{1 \ \text{ml}}{10 \ \text{gtt}} = 5 \ \text{ml/minute}$$

$$X = \frac{750 \ \text{ml}}{(50 \ \text{gtt/min} \div 10 \ \text{gtt/ml}) \times 60 \ \text{minutes}}$$

$$X = \frac{750}{5 \times 60 \ \text{hours}}$$

$$X = \frac{750 \ \text{ml}}{\dfrac{5 \ \text{ml}}{1 \ \text{min}} \times \dfrac{60 \ \text{min}}{1 \ \text{hour}}}$$

$$X = 2.5 \ \text{hours}$$

$$X = \frac{750}{300 \ \text{hours}}$$

> Congratulations! You've reached the peak of Mount I.V. Infusion!

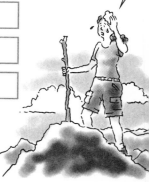

7

Special calculations

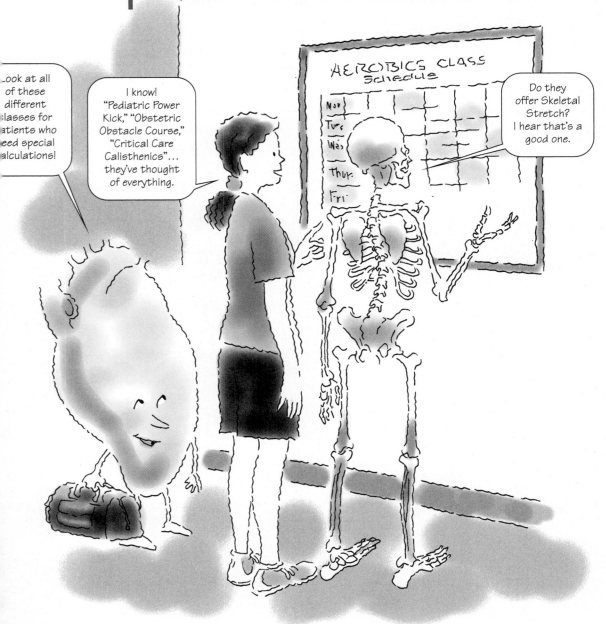

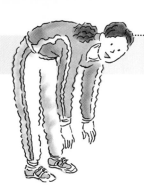

■ Warm-up

Special calculations review

Route guidelines

- P.O. medications may be given as liquid suspensions.
  - Mix the drug before measuring out dose.
  - Never crush timed-release capsules or tablets or enteric-coated drugs.
- SubQ is the route commonly used for childhood immunizations and insulin injections.
  - Make sure the injection contains no more than 1 ml of solution.
  - Administer in any area with sufficient subcutaneous tissue.
- I.M. is the route commonly used for vaccines.
  - Never inject more than 1 ml of solution in children.
  - Administer in the thigh of infants.
- I.V. drugs should be diluted carefully and administered cautiously.
  - Use an infusion pump for infants and small children.
- For topical route, absorption is greater in infants and small children.
  - Wipe off any remaining drug after application.
  - Apply according to practitioner's order and drug manufacturer's recommendations.

Dosages per kilogram

- Dosages are expressed as *mg/kg/day* or *mg/kg/dose*.
- Multiply the child's weight in kilograms by the required milligrams of drug per kilogram.

BSA

- Measured in m^2
- Determined through intersection of height and weight on a nomogram
- Multiplied by the prescribed dose in $mg/m^2/day$ to calculate safe pediatric dosages

Weight-based formulas for fluid needs

- A child weighing less than 10 kg:
weight in kg $\times$ 100 ml = fluid needs in ml/day
- A child weighing 10 to 20 kg:
(total kg – 10 kg) $\times$ 50 ml
- a child weighing more than 20 kg:
(total kg – 20 kg) $\times$ 20 ml = additional fluid need in ml/day;
1,500 ml/day + additional fluid need = fluid needs in ml/day

Calorie-based formula for fluid needs

- For a nondehydrated child:
fluid maintenance needs in ml/day =
BSA in $m^2 \times 1,500$ ml/day/m^2

Assessing the mother during drug administration

- Frequently check vital signs, urine output, uterine contractions, and deep tendon reflexes.
- Monitor and record fluid intake and output.
- Assess breath sounds.

Evaluating fetal response to drug therapy

- Monitor fetal heart rate during mother's drug therapy.
- If sudden increase or decrease occurs, immediately discontinue the drug.

Common obstetric drugs

Terbutaline

- Inhibits preterm labor
- Administered via an infusion pump and titrated every 10 minutes as needed

Magnesium sulfate

- Prevents or controls seizures caused by gestational hypertension
- Given as a loading dose first, then followed with infusion a lower dose
- Suspected toxicity requires stopping infusion immediately and notifying practitioner

Oxytocin

- Selectively stimulates uterine smooth muscle to induce labor
- May also be used to control bleeding after delivery of the placenta
- Administered I.V. piggyback with an infusion pump and titrated until normal contraction pattern occurs
- Requires careful monitoring of contraction strength

Dinoprostone

- Ripens the cervix (to induce labor) in pregnant patient at near term
- Available as endocervical gel, vaginal inserts, or vaginal suppositories

174

osage calculations

curate dosages of drugs given to the mother help avoid complications.
oportions can be used to solve obstetric dosage calcula-

alculating I.V. push dosages

e proportions to calculate dosages.
termine administration time.

alculating a drug's concentration

$$\text{centration in mg/ml} = \frac{\text{mg of drug}}{\text{ml of fluid}}$$

member to multiply the answer by 1,000 if you need to ess concentration in mcg/ml.

alculating the flow rate

r minute:

$$\frac{\text{minute}}{X} = \frac{\text{concentration of solution}}{1 \text{ ml of fluid}}$$

r hour:

$$\frac{\text{ly dose}}{X} = \frac{\text{concentration of solution}}{1 \text{ ml of fluid}}$$

Calculating a dosage in mg/kg of body weight/minute

- Determine the dose in milligrams per hour:
hourly flow rate × concentration
- Calculate the dose in milligrams per minute:
dose in mg/hour ÷ 60 minutes
- Solve for mg/kg/minute:
mg/minute ÷ patient's weight in kg

More formulas!

- To determine how many micrograms per kilogram per minute a patient is receiving:

$$\frac{\text{mg}}{\text{volume of bag}} \times 1{,}000 \div 60 \div \text{kg} \times \text{infusion rate} = \text{mcg/kg/minute}$$

- To determine how many milliliters per hour to give:

$$\frac{\text{weight in kg} \times \text{dose in mcg/kg/min} \times 60}{\text{concentration in 1 L}} = \text{ml/hr}$$

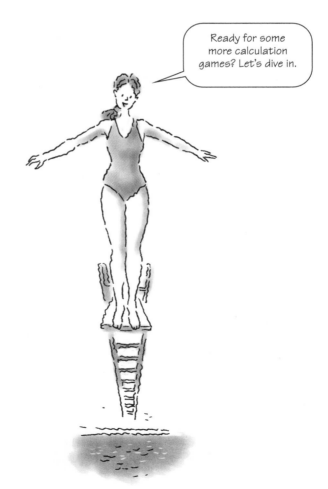

Ready for some more calculation games? Let's dive in.

■ Strikeout

Strike out the incorrect statements.

1. Drug administration for children is the same as it is for adults.

2. Children receive drugs via different routes than adults do.

3. Because of their immaturity, a child's body systems may be unable to handle certain drugs.

4. A child's total volume of body water is much greater proportionally than an adult's, so drug distribution is altered from an adult's.

5. An incorrect drug dose is more likely to harm an adult than a child.

6. Infants and children who can't swallow tablets or capsules are given oral drugs in liquid form.

7. When a liquid form of the drug isn't available, you should crush the tablet or capsule and put it in breast milk or infant formula.

8. You should never crush timed-release capsules or tablets or enteric-coated drugs.

9. If a child can't drink from a cup, you should use a medication dropper, syringe, or hollow-handle spoon.

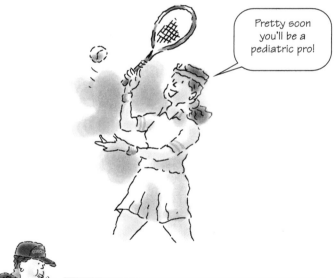

Pretty soon you'll be a pediatric pro!

Coaching session

Giving medications to children

Use these tips to guarantee safety when giving oral and parenteral medications to children.
- Check the child's mouth to be sure that he has swallowed an oral drug.
- Mix oral drugs that come in suspension form carefully.
- Use the vastus lateralis muscle to give I.M. injections in infants who haven't started walking.
- Rotate injection sites.

Match point

Match each administration route on the left with its corresponding description on the right.

Oral route _____

Subcutaneous route _____

I.M. route _____

I.V. route _____

Topical route _____

Options

A. Vaccines are commonly administered by this route.

B. Pediatric drugs administered via this route are diluted and administered cautiously because pediatric patients can tolerate only a limited amount of fluid.

C. When a liquid preparation isn't available, drugs administered by this route may generally be mixed with a small amount of liquid.

D. Absorption of drugs administered via this route is greater in pediatric patients than in adults because children have a greater ratio of total body surface area to weight.

E. Children may receive insulin via this route.

Hit or miss

Label each statement with a "T" for "True" or an "F" for "False."

_ 1. You should use a calculator to solve equations.

_ 2. When in doubt, you should ask a coworker to verify a drug dose.

_ 3. You should post the child's weight in kilograms at his bedside so that you won't have to estimate it or weigh him in a rush.

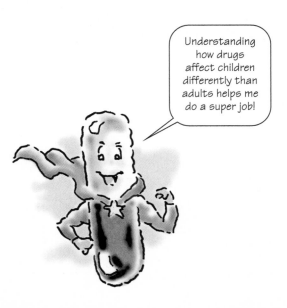

Understanding how drugs affect children differently than adults helps me do a super job!

Starting lineup

The practitioner orders a single dose of 20 mg/kg/dose of amoxicillin oral suspension for a toddler who weighs 20 lb (9.1
Put the following equation steps in the correct order to calculate the dose in milligrams.

$$X = 180 \text{ mg}$$

$$\frac{20 \text{ mg}}{1 \text{ kg/dose}} = \frac{X}{9 \text{ kg/dose}}$$

$$X \times \frac{\cancel{1 \text{ kg/dose}}}{\cancel{1 \text{ kg/dose}}} = 20 \text{ mg} \times \frac{9 \cancel{\text{ kg/dose}}}{1 \cancel{\text{ kg/dose}}}$$

$$X \times 1 \text{ kg/dose} = 20 \text{ mg} \times 9 \text{ kg/dose}$$

Be precise when you
calculate dosages. One mista
can send your pediatric clier
sliding downhill.

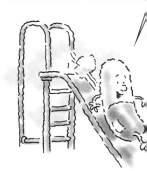

Dosage drills

Test your math skills with this drill.

Be sure to show
how you arrive at
your answer.

How many milligrams of a medication will a nurse give to a
32-lb child if the order calls for 25 mg/kg?

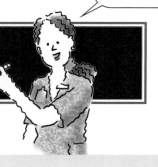

Your answer: _____

Match point

The practitioner orders penicillin V potassium oral suspension 50 mg/kg/day in four divided doses for a patient who weighs 44 lb. The suspension that's available is penicillin V potassium 150 mg/5ml. What volume should the nurse administer for each dose? Match the calculation sequence on the left with the correct equation(s) on the right.

Convert the child's weight from pounds to kilograms. _____

Multiply the means and the extremes. _____

Solve for X by dividing each side by 2.2 lb. _____

Determine the total daily dosage by setting up a proportion with the patient's weight and unknown dosage on one side and the ordered dosage on the other. _____

Cross-multiply the fractions. _____

Solve for X by dividing each side of the equation by 1 kg to determine the daily dose. _____

Divide the daily dosage by 4 doses to determine the dose to administer every 6 hours. _____

Calculate the volume to give for each dose by setting up a proportion with the unknown volume and the amount in one dose on one side and the available dose on the other. Cross-multiply the fractions. _____

Solve for X by dividing each side of the equation by 150 mg and canceling units that appear in both the numerator and denominator. _____

Options

A. $$\frac{X \times \cancel{1\,kg}}{\cancel{1\,kg}} = \frac{50\,mg \times 20\,\cancel{kg}}{1\,\cancel{kg}}$$

$$X = \frac{50\,mg \times 20\,kg}{1}$$

$$X = 1{,}000\,mg$$

B. $$X \times 2.2\,lb = 1\,kg \times 44\,lb$$

C. $$\frac{X}{250\,mg} = \frac{5\,ml}{150\,mg}$$

$$X \times 150\,mg = 5\,ml \times 250\,mg$$

D. $$X : 44\,lb :: 1\,kg : 2.2\,lb$$

E. $$X = \frac{1{,}000\,mg}{4\,doses}$$

$$X = 250\,mg/dose$$

F. $$\frac{X \times \cancel{2.2\,lb}}{\cancel{2.2\,lb}} = \frac{1\,kg \times 44\,\cancel{lb}}{2.2\,\cancel{lb}}$$

$$X = \frac{44\,kg}{2.2}$$

$$X = 20\,kg$$

G. $$X \times 1\,kg = 50\,mg \times 20\,kg$$

H. $$X \times \frac{\cancel{150\,mg}}{\cancel{150\,mg}} = \frac{5\,ml \times 250\,\cancel{mg}}{150\,\cancel{mg}}$$

$$X \times \frac{5\,ml \times 250}{150}$$

$$X = \frac{1{,}250\,mg}{150}$$

$$X = 8.3\,ml$$

I. $$\frac{20\,kg}{X} = \frac{1\,kg}{50\,mg}$$

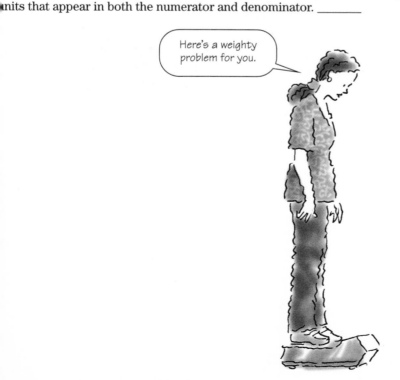

Here's a weighty problem for you.

■■
■ Batter's box

Fill in the blanks with the correct answer options in this formula about how to calculate a child's dose based on the average adult BSA—1.73 m²—and an average adult dose.

$$\text{child's dose in mg} = \frac{(1)}{(2)} \times \boxed{(3)}$$

> **Options**
>
> A. child's BSA in m^2
>
> B. average adult dose
>
> C. average adult BSA (1.73 m^2)

■■
■ Dosage drills

Test your math skills with this drill.

> Be sure to show how you arrive at your answer.

A patient with gestational hypertension is receiving 8 g of magnesium sulfate in 1 L of dextrose 5% in water at 125 ml/hr. How many grams per hour is the patient receiving?

Your answer: _____

Match point

Use the nomogram on this page to match the measurements on the left with the appropriate measurement on the right.

	Options
Height = 60 in; surface area = 0.7 m² _____	A. Surface area = 0.53 m²
Height = 70 cm; weight = 40 lbs _____	B. Height = 57 in
Surface area = 1.0 m²; weight = 28 kg _____	C. Weight = 21 lbs

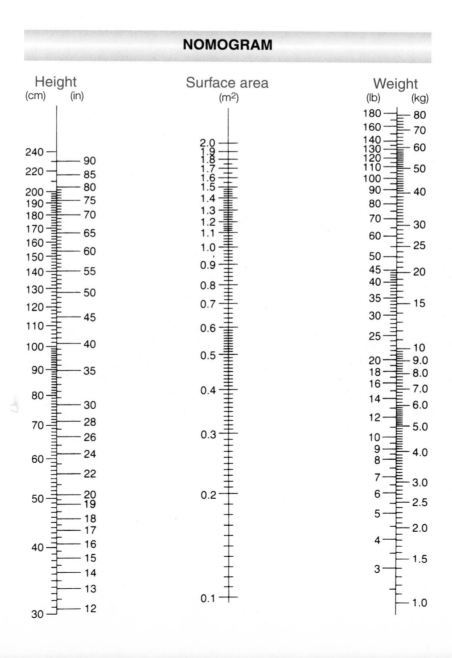

NOMOGRAM

■■
■ Batter's box

Fill in the blanks with the correct information regarding the body surface area (BSA) method.

To calculate dosage by BSA, plot the patient's _____ and
                                                    1

_____ on a _____ . Then multiply the BSA by
        2   3

the prescribed pediatric dose in _____ .
                                          4

> When it comes to verifying correct dosage, nurses run defense. We're the last line of defense to ensure that the ordered dosage is safe.

Options

A. nomogram

B. $mg/m^2/day$

C. weight

D. height

■■
■ Dosage drills

Test your math skills with this drill.

> Be sure to show how you arrive at your answer.

A pediatric patient who weighs 44 lbs (20 kg) is to receive erythromycin for bronchitis at 15 mg/kg in each dose. How many milligrams should the nurse administer?

Your answer: _____

Starting lineup

A child who needs chemotherapy is 38″ tall and weighs 35 lb. Arrange the following steps in the correct order to calculate the safe drug dose in milligrams if the average adult dose is 1,000 mg.

Solve for X by canceling units that appear in both the numerator and denominator, multiplying the child's BSA by the average adult dose, and dividing the result by the average adult BSA:

$$X = \frac{0.66 \; \cancel{m^2} \times 1,000 \; mg}{1.73 \; \cancel{m^2}}$$

$$X = 381.5 \; mg$$

Set up an equation using the appropriate formula. Divide the child's BSA by 1.73 m² (the average adult BSA), and multiply by the average adult dose, 1,000 mg:

$$X = \frac{0.66 \; \cancel{m^2}}{1.73 \; \cancel{m^2}} \times 1,000 \; mg$$

Use the nomogram to determine that the child's BSA is 0.66 m².

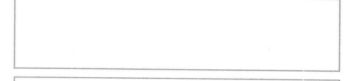

If you're feeling a bit shaky on all these dosage calculations, remember: Practice makes perfect!

Match point

The practitioner orders chloral hydrate 125 mg P.O. to sedate a 5-kg neonate for an electroencephalogram. The drug handbook states that the usual (recommended) dosage of chloral hydrate for a neonate is 25 mg/kg/dose for sedation prior to a procedure. Match the calculation sequence on the left with the correct equation on the right to verify that the ordered dosage is correct.

Options

Set up the proportion with the usual dosage in one fraction and the unknown dosage and the patient's weight in the other fraction. _____

Cross-multiply the fractions. _____

Solve for X by dividing each side of the equation by 1 kg/dose and canceling units that appear in both the numerator and denominator. _____

Check the result. _____

A. $\dfrac{X \times \cancel{1\,kg/dose}}{\cancel{1\,kg/dose}} = \dfrac{25\,mg \times 5\,\cancel{kg/dose}}{1\,\cancel{kg/dose}}$

B. $X = 125\,mg$

C. $\dfrac{25\,mg}{1\,kg/dose} = \dfrac{X}{5\,kg/dose}$

D. $X \times 1\,kg/dose = 25\,mg \times 5\,kg/dose$

■ A-maze-ing race

The practitioner orders penicillin V potassium oral suspension 200 mg P.O. q6h for a patient who weighs 44 lb. The medication is available as 125 mg/5 ml. Is the dose safe? Identify the correct numerical calculation sequence while you power walk through this maze and then treat yourself to a massage.

1. First, convert the child's weight from pounds to kilograms using a proportion.

2. Multiply the extremes and the means.

3. Solve for X by dividing each side of the equation by 2.2 lb and canceling units th
   appear in both the numerator and denominator to determine the child's weight.

4. Now verify the usual (recommended) dosage. The drug reference says to give penicillin V potassium 25 to 50 mg/kg/day orally in divided doses every 6 to 8 ho
   This indicates a safe daily dosage range—a low dosage (25 mg/kg/day) and a hi
   dosage (50 mg/kg/day). Next, determine the usual total daily dosage range by se
   up two proportions with the patient's weight on one side and the usual dosage
   the other. Use the high dosage first.

5. Cross-multiply the fractions.

6. Solve for X to determine the child's maximum daily dosage.

7. Now divide the daily dosage by four doses to determine the maximum safe dos
   administer every 6 hours.

8. Repeat the same steps (set up the proportion, cross-multiply the fractions, and
   solve for X) to determine the low or minimum dose.

9. Divide the daily dosage by four doses to determine the minimum safe dose to administer every 6 hours.

10. Calculate the volume to give for each dose by setting up a proportion with the unknown volume and the amount in one dose on one side and the available dos
    the other side.

11. Solve for X.

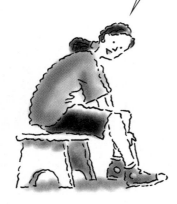

Lace up your running shoes and follow me. We'll get through this maze in no time.

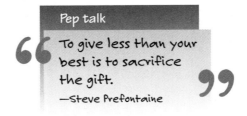

Pep talk

" To give less than your best is to sacrifice the gift.
—Steve Prefontaine "

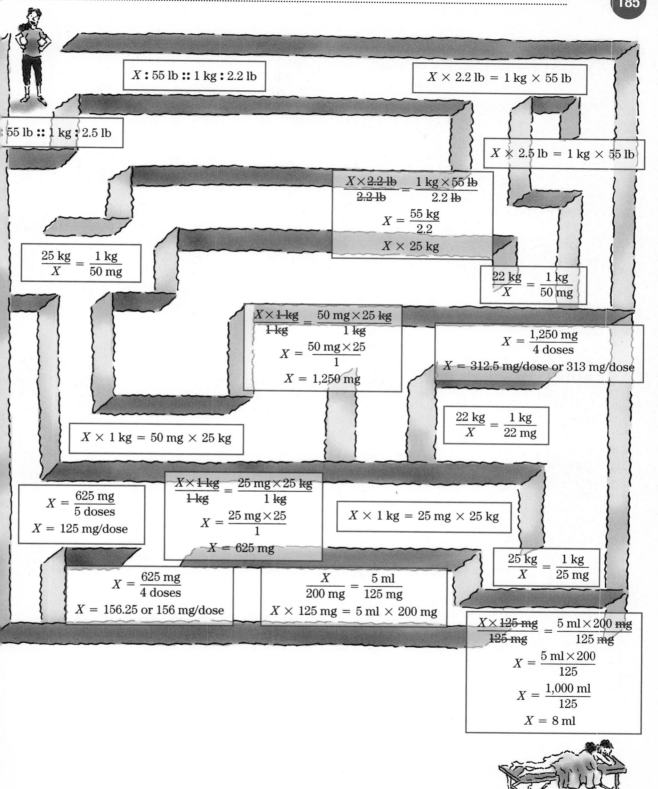

$X : 55\text{ lb} :: 1\text{ kg} : 2.2\text{ lb}$

$X \times 2.2\text{ lb} = 1\text{ kg} \times 55\text{ lb}$

$55\text{ lb} :: 1\text{ kg} : 2.5\text{ lb}$

$X \times 2.5\text{ lb} = 1\text{ kg} \times 55\text{ lb}$

$$\frac{X \times 2.2\text{ lb}}{2.2\text{ lb}} = \frac{1\text{ kg} \times 55\text{ lb}}{2.2\text{ lb}}$$
$$X = \frac{55\text{ kg}}{2.2}$$
$$X \times 25\text{ kg}$$

$$\frac{25\text{ kg}}{X} = \frac{1\text{ kg}}{50\text{ mg}}$$

$$\frac{22\text{ kg}}{X} = \frac{1\text{ kg}}{50\text{ mg}}$$

$$\frac{X \times 1\text{ kg}}{1\text{ kg}} = \frac{50\text{ mg} \times 25\text{ kg}}{1\text{ kg}}$$
$$X = \frac{50\text{ mg} \times 25}{1}$$
$$X = 1{,}250\text{ mg}$$

$$X = \frac{1{,}250\text{ mg}}{4\text{ doses}}$$
$$X = 312.5\text{ mg/dose or } 313\text{ mg/dose}$$

$X \times 1\text{ kg} = 50\text{ mg} \times 25\text{ kg}$

$$\frac{22\text{ kg}}{X} = \frac{1\text{ kg}}{22\text{ mg}}$$

$$X = \frac{625\text{ mg}}{5\text{ doses}}$$
$$X = 125\text{ mg/dose}$$

$$\frac{X \times 1\text{ kg}}{1\text{ kg}} = \frac{25\text{ mg} \times 25\text{ kg}}{1\text{ kg}}$$
$$X = \frac{25\text{ mg} \times 25}{1}$$
$$X = 625\text{ mg}$$

$X \times 1\text{ kg} = 25\text{ mg} \times 25\text{ kg}$

$$\frac{25\text{ kg}}{X} = \frac{1\text{ kg}}{25\text{ mg}}$$

$$X = \frac{625\text{ mg}}{4\text{ doses}}$$
$$X = 156.25 \text{ or } 156\text{ mg/dose}$$

$$\frac{X}{200\text{ mg}} = \frac{5\text{ ml}}{125\text{ mg}}$$
$$X \times 125\text{ mg} = 5\text{ ml} \times 200\text{ mg}$$

$$\frac{X \times 125\text{ mg}}{125\text{ mg}} = \frac{5\text{ ml} \times 200\text{ mg}}{125\text{ mg}}$$
$$X = \frac{5\text{ ml} \times 200}{125}$$
$$X = \frac{1{,}000\text{ ml}}{125}$$
$$X = 8\text{ ml}$$

■ Starting lineup

Put these steps in the order needed to start a continuous infusion.

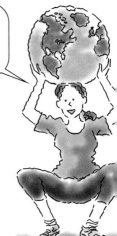

Now try these exercises for a real-world workout in verifying calculations.

Mix the drug thoroughly.

Calculate the dosage.

Label the I.V. bag or fluid chamber with the drug's name, the dosage, the time and date it was mixed, and your initials.

Draw up the drug in a syringe; then add the drug to the I.V. bag or fluid chamber through the drug additive port, using aseptic technique.

Hang the solution and administer the drug by infusion pump at the prescribed flow rate.

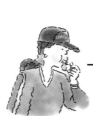

Coaching session

Continuous infusions

Continuous infusions are used for pediatric patients who require around-the-clock fluids, drug therapy, or both. To prepare for a continuous drug infusion, add the drug to a small-volume bag of I.V. fluid or a volume-control device. Mix the solution carefully according to the manufacturer's guidelines.

In most cases, a volume-control device, such as a small-volume bag of I.V. fluid with a microdrip set or a Buretrol set, maintains the flow rate by using a positive-pressure pumping mechanism. Such a device is used for continuous and intermittent infusion because accurate fluid administration is extremely important for pediatric patients. Remember: Pediatric patients can tolerate only small amounts of fluid.

Jumble gym

Fill in the blank letters in the statements below and then use these letters to make the word that completes this sentence:

tion: The rate of I.V. infusion must be carefully controlled to ensure proper _____ and to
ent or minimize toxicity associated with rapid infusion.

Volume-con__rol devices are c__librated in 1-ml __ncrements.

ntermittent infu__ion is commonly used in acute and h__me care settings.

Medication-filled syringes with microtu__ing can be used to i__fuse small volumes via syringe __umps.

Accuracy is especially imp__rtant with pediat__ic patients.

er: __ __ __ __ __ __ __ __ __ __

> You're up!
> Let's see you
> take a swing at
> putting these
> steps in order.

Starting lineup

Arrange these steps in the correct order for the procedure of starting an intermittent
nfusion using a volume-control device.

Draw up the prescribed volume of drug into the syringe.	
Label the volume-control device with the name of the drug.	
Add the drug to the fluid chamber through the drug additive port.	
Disconnect the device when the flush is complete.	
Carefully calculate the prescribed volume of drug.	
Mix the drug thoroughly.	
culate the appropriate flow rate and infuse the drug.	
Attach the volume-control device to an electronic infusion pump to control the infusion rate.	
Flush the line to clear the tubing of the drug.	

See how quickly you can run this drill. Ready, set, go!

■■ Dosage drills

Test your math skills with this drill.

Be sure to show how you arrive at your answer.

> The average adult dose of codeine phosphate for pain is 60 mg P.O. every 4 hours. How much should a nurse administer in a single dose to a child with a body surface area of 0.55 m²?

Your answer: _____

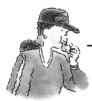

Coaching session
Calculating pediatric fluids

You can calculate the number of milliliters of fluid a child needs based on three different factors:
- the child's weight in kilograms
- metabolism (calories required)
- BSA in square meters.

Remember: Fluid replacement can also be affected by clinical conditions that cause fluid retention or loss, so children with these conditions should receive fluids based on their individual needs.

Strikeout

Strike out the equation that doesn't help solve this problem.

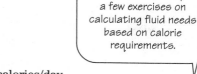

Now let's serve up a few exercises on calculating fluid needs based on calorie requirements.

Question: Your pediatric patient weighs 24 lbs and uses 1100 calories/day. What are his daily fluid requirements?

$$\frac{24\ \text{lb}}{X} = \frac{100\ \text{kcal}}{1100\ \text{kcal}}$$

$$X = \frac{1{,}100\ \cancel{\text{kcal}}}{100\ \cancel{\text{kcal}}} \times 120\ \text{ml}$$

$$X = 11 \times 120\ \text{ml}$$

$$X = 1{,}320\ \text{ml}$$

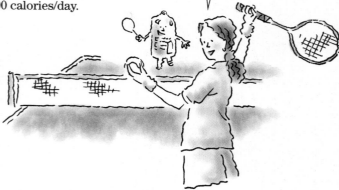

Batter's box

Fill in the blanks with the correct answer options in this equation to determine fluid needs based on calorie requirements.

$$\text{d needs in}\ \boxed{(1)} = \frac{\boxed{(2)}\ \text{requirements}}{100\ \text{kcal}} \times \boxed{(3)}\ \text{ml}$$

Options

A. 120

B. calorie

C. ml/day

Pep talk

" Being the first to cross the finish line makes you a winner in only one phase of life. It's what you do after you cross the line that really counts. "

—Ralph Boston

Match point

How much fluid should you give a 55-lb patient over 24 hours to meet his maintenance needs? Match the calculation sequence on the left to the correct equation(s) on the right.

Clues

1. Convert 55 lb to kilograms by setting up a proportion with fractions. _____

2. Cross-multiply the fractions and then solve for X by dividing both sides of the equation by 2.2 lb. _____

3. Subtract 10 kg from the child's weight and multiply the result by 50 ml/kg/day to find the child's additional fluid need. _____

4. Add the additional fluid need to the 1,000 ml/day required for the first 10 kg. _____

Options

A. $\dfrac{55\ lb}{X} = \dfrac{2.2\ lb}{1\ kg}$

B. $X = (25\ kg - 10\ kg) \times 50\ ml/kg/da$
$X = 15\ kg \times 50\ ml/kg/day$
$X = 750\ ml/day\ additional\ fluid\ ne$

C. $X \times 2.2\ lb = 55\ lb \times 1\ kg$
$\dfrac{X \times 2.2\ lb}{2.2\ lb} = \dfrac{55\ lb \times 1\ kg}{2.2\ lb}$
$X = \dfrac{55\ kg}{2.2}$
$X = 25\ kg$

D. $X = 1,000\ ml/day + 750\ ml/day$
$X = 1,750\ ml/day$

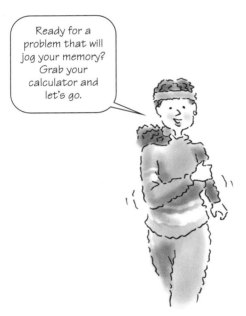

Ready for a problem that will jog your memory? Grab your calculator and let's go.

Hit or miss

Label each statement with a "T" for "True" or an "F" for "False."

_____ 1. Body surface area (BSA) is determined by setting up a proportion where every pound of the child's weight is multiplied by 2.2.

_____ 2. To calculate the daily fluid needs of a child who isn't dehydrated, you should multiply the BSA by 1,100.

_____ 3. The daily fluid needs of a patient who is 38″ tall, weighs 42 lb (19 kg), and has a BSA of 0.75 m^2 are 1,110 m

_____ 4. BSA is multiplied by the prescribed dose in mg/m^2/day to calculate safe pediatric dosages.

Dosage drills

Test your math skills with this drill.

> Be sure to show how you arrive at your answer.

A 52-lb (23.6-kg) child receives 5 mg/kg of phenytoin (Dilantin) for seizure control in two divided doses. The bottle contains a concentration of 125 mg/5 ml. How many milliliters per dose should the nurse instruct the parent to administer?

Your answer: _____

Match point

The practitioner orders a single dose of 550 mg of ampicillin for an infant who weighs 12 lb. The usual (recommended) dose is 100 mg/kg/dose. The ampicillin is available in a concentration of 500 mg/5 ml. What volume of ampicillin should you administer? Match the calculation sequence on the left to the correct answer on the right.

Verify that the ordered dose is correct by setting up a proportion to determine the child's weight in kilograms. Cross-multiply the fractions and solve for X. _____

Set up a proportion with the recommended dosage in one fraction and the unknown dosage and the patient's weight in the other. Cross-multiply the fractions and solve for X. _____

Determine the volume of drug to administer by setting up a proportion with the known concentration in one fraction and the desired dose and unknown volume in the other fraction. Cross-multiply the fractions and solve for X. _____

Options

A. $X = 545$ mg

B. $X = 5.5$ ml

C. $X = 5.45$ kg

Cross-training

Here's an exercise to pump up your knowledge of pediatric drug administration.

Across

1. P.O. medication may be given as _____ suspensions.

4. A _____ set is a volume-control device.

7. You should never _____ timed-release capsules.

8. A _____ plots height and weight to determine body surface area.

10. Route commonly used for insulin injections

12. I.V. drugs should be _____ carefully.

Down

2. I.V. drugs can be administered by continuous or _____ infusion.

3. You can calculate fluid needs based on these.

5. _____ is measured in M^2.

6. Route commonly used for vaccines.

9. Children's fluid needs are proportionally _____ than those of adults.

11. 120 ml per 100 kcal is the _____-to-calorie ratio.

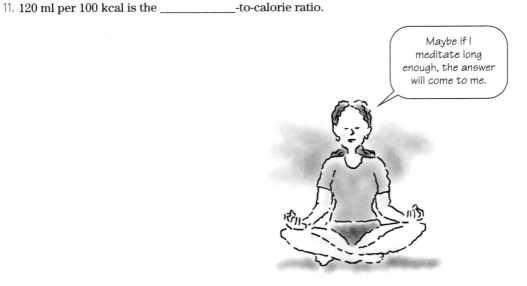

Maybe if I meditate long enough, the answer will come to me.

Strikeout

Drugs are commonly given during pregnancy, labor and delivery, and the postpartum period for four reasons. Strike out the incorrect reasons.

To control gestational hypertension

To improve renal function

To minimize maternal weight gain

To inhibit preterm labor

To support fetal growth

To induce labor

To prevent postpartum hemorrhage

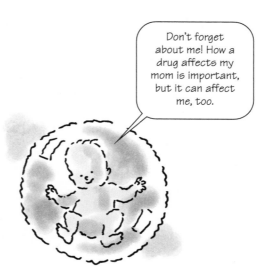

Don't forget about me! How a drug affects my mom is important, but it can affect me, too.

Batter's box

Fill in the blanks with the correct information regarding assessment of fetal heart tones during drug therapy.

tantly assess fetal heart tones and heart _____ by connecting the
                                                    1

er to an electronic _____ monitor. Be alert for a sudden increase or
                                2

_____ in fetal heart rate, which may signal an _____
        3   4

_____ to treatment. If either occurs, _____ drug treatment
        5   6

diately.

Options

A. fetal

B. reaction

C. discontinue

D. rate

E. decrease

F. adverse

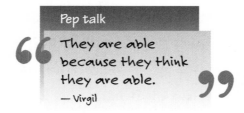

Pep talk

They are able because they think they are able.
— Virgil

Hit or miss

The drugs used most commonly during pregnancy, labor and delivery, and the postpartum period are terbutaline (Brethin magnesium sulfate, dinoprostone (Cervidil), and oxytocin (Pitocin). Label each statement about these drugs with a "T" for "True" or an "F" for "False."

_____ 1. Terbutaline is used to inhibit preterm labor. You should mix it in a compatible I.V. solution and administer it through an infusion pump.

_____ 2. Dinoprostone should be used cautiously in labor and in those with impaired renal function, myocardial damage, or heart block.

_____ 3. Oxytocin can be administered by piggyback infusion so the drug can be discontinued without interrupting the I.V. line.

_____ 4. Magnesium sulfate is contraindicated in cephalopelvic disproportion, fetal distress, and other obstetric emergencies.

_____ 5. Terbutaline relaxes the uterine muscle by acting on beta$_2$-adrenergic receptors.

_____ 6. Dinoprostone can cause adverse reactions in the fetus that include hyperstimulation, respiratory depression, and bradycardia.

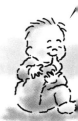

Someday I'll be an athlete, but right now my on workout is sucki on my toes.

> ❝ The concept of total wellness recognizes that our every thought, word, and behavior affects our greater health and well-being. And we, in turn, are affected not only emotionally but also physically and spiritually. ❞
> —Greg Anderson

Pep talk

Jumble gym

Fill in the blank letters in the statements below and then use these letters to make the word that completes this sentence

Question: Oxytocin may be used to control bleeding after delivery of the _____.

1. Magnesium sulfate prevents or controls seizures that may be caused by gestational hy__ertension.

2. Dinoprostone is available as an __ __docervical ge__ or a v__ginal insert or suppository.

3. After labor is established, the doctor may decrease the infusion r__te of oxy__ocin.

4. When administering dinoprostone, have the patient lie on her ba__k.

Answer: __ __ __ __ __ __ __ __

Match point

The practitioner orders oxytocin to stimulate labor for a woman who is 10 days overdue. The order reads *1 ml (10 units) oxytocin in 1 L (1,000 ml) NSS; infuse via pump at 2 milliunits/minute for 20 minutes and then increase flow rate to 3 milliunits/minute.* What's the solution's concentration? What's the flow rate needed to deliver 2 milliunits/minute for 20 minutes? What's the flow rate needed to deliver 3 milliunits/minute thereafter? Match the calculation sequence on the top with the correct equation(s) on the bottom.

Cues

1. Determine the concentration of the solution. Cross-multiply the fractions and solve for *X*. _____

2. Determine the flow rate. Cross-multiply the fractions and solve for *X*. _____

3. Calculate the flow rate to be used after the first 20 minutes. Cross-multiply the fractions and solve for *X*. _____

Options

$$\frac{2 \text{ milliunits}}{1 \text{ minute}} \times 20 \text{ minutes} = 40 \text{ milliunits}$$

$$\frac{10 \text{ milliunits}}{1 \text{ ml}} = \frac{40 \text{ milliunits}}{X}$$

$$X \times 10 \text{ milliunits} = 1 \text{ ml} \times 40 \text{ milliunits}$$

$$\frac{X \times \cancel{10 \text{ milliunits}}}{\cancel{10 \text{ milliunits}}} = \frac{1 \text{ ml} \times 40 \cancel{\text{ milliunits}}}{10 \cancel{\text{ milliunits}}}$$

$$X = \frac{40 \text{ ml}}{10}$$

$$X = 4 \text{ ml in 20 minutes}$$

$$\frac{4 \text{ ml}}{20 \text{ minutes}} = \frac{X \text{ ml}}{60 \text{ minutes}}$$

$$4 \text{ ml} \times 60 \text{ minutes} = X \text{ ml} \times 20 \text{ minutes}$$

$$\frac{4 \text{ ml} \times 60 \cancel{\text{ minutes}}}{20 \cancel{\text{ minutes}}} = \frac{X \text{ ml} \times 20 \cancel{\text{ minutes}}}{20 \cancel{\text{ minutes}}}$$

$$X \text{ ml} = \frac{240 \text{ ml}}{20}$$

$$X = 12 \text{ ml/hour}$$

B.
$$\frac{10 \text{ milliunits}}{1 \text{ ml}} = \frac{180 \text{ milliunits}}{X}$$

$$X \times 10 \text{ milliunits} = 1 \text{ ml} \times 180 \text{ milliunits}$$

$$\frac{X \times \cancel{10 \text{ milliunits}}}{\cancel{10 \text{ milliunits}}} = \frac{1 \text{ ml} \times 180 \cancel{\text{ milliunits}}}{10 \cancel{\text{ milliunits}}}$$

$$X = \frac{180 \text{ ml}}{10}$$

$$X = 18 \text{ ml/hour}$$

C.
$$\frac{10 \text{ units}}{1,000 \text{ ml}} = \frac{X}{1 \text{ ml}}$$

$$X \times 1,000 \text{ ml} = 10 \text{ units} \times 1 \text{ ml}$$

$$\frac{X \times \cancel{1,000 \text{ ml}}}{\cancel{1,000 \text{ ml}}} = \frac{10 \text{ units} \times 1 \cancel{\text{ ml}}}{1,000 \cancel{\text{ ml}}}$$

$$X = \frac{10 \text{ units}}{1,000}$$

$$X = 0.01 \text{ unit or 10 milliunits/ml}$$

■■
■ Dosage drills

Test your math skills with this drill.

> Be sure to show how you arrive at your answer.

> A patient is in preterm labor. The practitioner prescribes 10 mg terbutaline sulfate in 250 ml D$_5$W to infuse at 5 mcg/minute. What's the flow rate for the solution?

Your answer: _____

■■
■ Starting lineup

Your patient is at risk for a seizure due to gestational hypertension. The practitioner orders *8 g (8,000 mg) magnesium sulfa* *in 500 ml D$_5$W to be infused at 2 g/hour.* Put these steps in the correct order to calculate the flow rate in milliliters per hour

Calculate the flow rate by setting up another proportion with the solution concentration in one fraction and the unknown flow rate in the other fraction. Cross-multiply the fractions and solve for *X*.	
Cross-multiply the fractions.	
Solve for *X* by dividing each side of the equation by 500 ml.	
Calculate the strength of the solution by setting up a proportion with the known strength in one fraction and the unknown strength in the other fraction.	

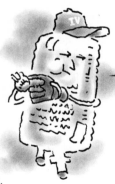

Let's see if you can pitch one over the plate by completing this crossword puzzle in record time!

Cross-training

Here's an exercise to expand your knowledge of obstetric drug dosages.

Across

1. If sudden increases or decreases in fetal heart rate occur, _____ the drug.

4. Dinoprostone is available as an endocervical _____.

7. When administering maternal medications, you should check vital signs, urine output, contractions, and deep _____ reflexes.

8. Oxytocin stimulates _____ smooth muscle.

Down

1. Dinoprostone induces labor by _____ the cervix.

2. Terbutaline is administered via _____.

3. Magnesium sulfate prevents or controls _____.

5. _____ may be used to control bleeding after delivery of the placenta.

6. _____ inhibits preterm labor.

9. Accurate drug dosages given to the mother help avoid _____ complications.

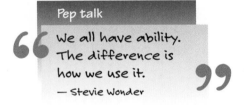

Pep talk

We all have ability. The difference is how we use it.

— Stevie Wonder

Train your brain

Solve this riddle to reveal a statement about dosage calculations.

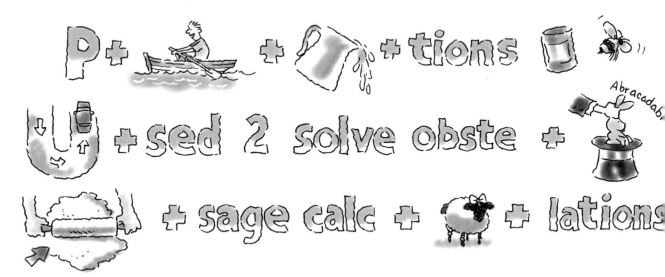

Jumble gym

Fill in the blank letters in the statements below and then use these letters to make the word that completes this sentence:

Question: **Many drugs administered on critical care units are given by direct injection, also called** _____.

1. Many I.__. drugs are administered in life-threatening situations.

2. On a critical care unit, you need to perform do__age calc__lations quickly.

3. The nurse's job is to __repare the drug for __nfusion, give it to the patient, and then observe __im to evaluate the drug's effectiveness.

Answer: __ __ __ __ __ __

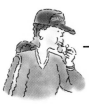

These four tips get rid of more stress than a round of golf does. Fore!

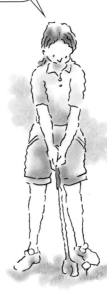

Coaching session
Subverting stress

Working in critical care can be stressful, especially when you must calculate dosages during an emergency. Being stressed means you may be more likely to make a mistake. To help you make quick and accurate dosage calculations during an emergency, be prepared by keeping these four tips in mind:

Keep a list of all the drug-calculation formulas in your pocket.

Carry a calculator.

Convert your patients' weights into kilograms and keep this information at their bedsides.

Become familiar with your unit's medication protocols and the most common critical care I.V. drugs.

Match point

Your patient is admitted with frequent ventricular arrhythmias. The practitioner orders procainamide 200 mg q5 min by slow I.V. push (no faster than 25 to 50 mg/minute) until arrhythmias disappear. If the drug label says the dose strength is 100 mg/ml, how many milliliters of procainamide should you give to the patient every 5 minutes? Match the calculation sequence on the left with the correct equation(s) on the right.

es

. Set up a proportion with the ordered dose and the unknown volume in one fraction and the dose strength in milligrams per milliliter in the other fraction. _____

. Cross-multiply the fractions. _____

. Solve for X by dividing each side of the equation by 100 mg and canceling the units that appear in both the numerator and denominator. _____

Options

A. $X \times 100 \text{ mg} = 1 \text{ ml} \times 200 \text{ mg}$

B. $\dfrac{200 \text{ mg}}{X} = \dfrac{100 \text{ mg}}{1 \text{ ml}}$

C. $\dfrac{X \times \cancel{100 \text{ mg}}}{\cancel{100 \text{ mg}}} = \dfrac{1 \text{ ml} \times 200 \cancel{\text{ mg}}}{100 \cancel{\text{ mg}}}$

$X = \dfrac{200 \text{ ml}}{100}$

$X = 2 \text{ ml}$

Dosage drills

Test your math skills with this drill.

> Be sure to show how you arrive at your answer.

A patient with supraventricular tachycardia is ordered esmolol hydrocholride (Brevibloc) at 50 mcg/kg/minute. The solution contains 2.5 g esmolol in 250 ml of D₅W. The patient weighs 73 kg. How should the nurse set the pump to deliver the correct milliliters per hour so the patient receives the ordered dose?

Your answer: _____

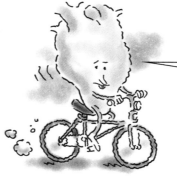

> Don't just sit there—get up and do something! I hope I'm not the only one getting a workout here!

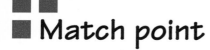

Match point

Match each drug with its correct unit of measurement. Note that options will be used more than once.

Clues

1. Procainamide _____
2. Epinephrine _____
3. Phenylephrine _____
4. Nitroglycerin _____
5. Nitroprusside _____
6. Lidocaine _____
7. Dobutamine _____

Options

A. mcg/kg/minute
B. mcg/minute
C. mg/minute

Pep talk

"The greater the difficulty, the more glory in surmounting it.
—Epictetus"

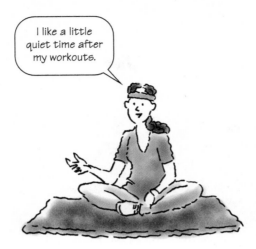

Batter's box

Before administering critical care drugs, you may need to perform three types of calculations. Fill in the blanks with the correct information regarding these calculations.

_____ of the drug in the I.V. solution

_____ rate required to deliver the desired dose

Number of _____ needed, based on the patient's weight in kilograms

Options

A. micrograms

B. concentration

C. flow

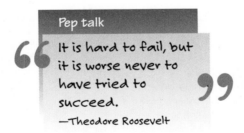

Pep talk

It is hard to fail, but it is worse never to have tried to succeed.

—Theodore Roosevelt

Hit or miss

Label each statement with a "T" for "True" or an "F" for "False."

___ 1. To calculate an I.V. push dosage, you should use proportions to calculate the dosage.

___ 2. When calculating a dosage in mg/kg of body weight/minute, you should multiply the hourly flow rate by 1,000 to determine the dose in milligrams per hour.

___ 3. If you need to express a concentration in mcg/ml (instead of mg/ml), you should multiply by 100.

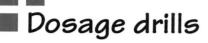

Dosage drills

Test your math skills with this drill.

> Be sure to show how you arrive at your answer.

A patient weighing 106 kg has an order for 5 mcg/kg/minute of dobutamine (Dobutrex). The concentration is 500 mg dobutamine in 250 ml of D₅W. How should the nurse set the pump to deliver the correct infusion rate?

Your answer: _____

Coaching session
Card-carrying calculation

> Keeping my life in balance helps me manage stress and be more productive at my job.

Working with critical care patients, you may encounter situations in which you don't have time to refer to your dosage calculation book. If you keep these formulas on a card with your calculator for quick reference, you won't miss a beat.

• To determine how many micrograms per kilogram per minute your patient is receiving, use this formula:

$$\text{mcg/kg/minute} = \frac{\text{mg}}{\text{volume of bag}} \times 1{,}000 \div 60 \div \text{kg} \times \text{infusion rate}$$

• To determine how many milliliters per hour you should give, use this formula:

$$\text{ml/hr} = \frac{\text{weight in kg} \times \text{dose in mcg/kg/minute} \times 60}{\text{concentration in 1L}}$$

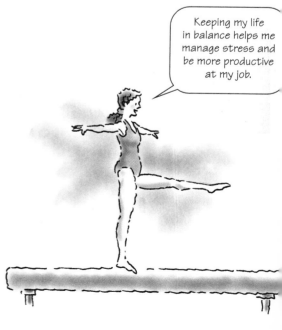

SPECIAL CALCULATIONS

203

Match point

Your patient is having frequent runs of ventricular tachycardia that subside after 10 to 12 beats. The practitioner orders *2g (2,000 mg) lidocaine in 500 ml D₅W to infuse at 2 mg/minute.* What's the flow rate in milliliters per minute? In milliliters per hour? Match the sequence of calculations on the left with the *X* value on the right.

ues

1. First, find the solution's concentration by setting up a proportion with the unknown concentration in one fraction and the ordered dose in the other. Cross-multiply the fractions and solve for *X*. _____

2. Next, calculate the flow rate per minute needed to deliver the ordered dose of 2 mg/minute by setting up a proportion with the unknown flow rate per minute in one fraction and the solution's concentration in the other. Cross-multiply the fractions and solve for *X*. _____

3. Compute the hourly flow rate by setting up a proportion with the unknown flow rate per hour in one fraction and the flow rate per minute in the other. Cross-multiply the fractions and solve for *X*. _____

Options

A. $X = 0.5$ ml

B. $X = 30$ ml

C. $X = 4$ mg

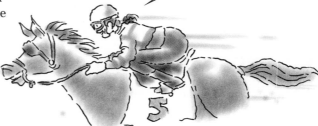

Speed matters. In nursing critical care patients, you need to perform dosage calculations accurately AND quickly.

Dosage drills

Test your math skills with this drill.

Be sure to show how you arrive at your answer.

A patient with heart failure has a solution containing 20 mg of milrinone (Primacor) in 200 ml of D5W infusing at 20 ml/hr. The patient weighs 90 kg. What dose is the patient receiving in micrograms per kilogram per minute?

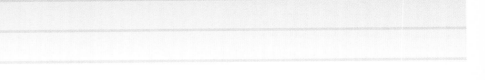

Your answer: _____

Batter's box

Fill in the blanks with the correct information in this equation to calculate a drug's concentration.

Concentration in [(1)] $= \dfrac{(2)}{(3)}$

Options

A. ml of fluid

B. mg of drug

C. mg/ml

If I concentrate, I can do anything!

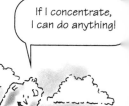

Starting lineup

A patient with terminal Hodgkin's disease who weighs 90 lb (41 kg) has been hypotensive for several hours despite receiving I.V. fluid boluses. The practitioner orders 200 mg phenylephrine in 500 ml of normal saline solution. The drug is to start at 25 mcg/minute and then be titrated to keep the systolic blood pressure at 90 mm Hg. Put the following equation steps in the correct order to calculate the flow rate in milliliters per minute.

$$0.4 \text{ mg/ml} \times 1{,}000 = 400 \text{ mcg/ml}$$

$$\frac{25 \text{ mcg/minute}}{X \text{ ml/minute}} = \frac{400 \text{ mcg}}{1 \text{ ml}}$$

$$\frac{X \text{ ml/minute} \times \cancel{400 \text{ mcg}}}{\cancel{400 \text{ mcg}}} = \frac{25 \cancel{\text{ mcg}}/\text{minute} \times 1 \text{ ml}}{\cancel{400 \text{ mcg}}}$$

$$X = \frac{25 \text{ ml/minute}}{400}$$

$$X = 0.0625 \text{ ml/minute}$$

$$X \text{ ml/minute} \times 400 \text{ mcg} = 25 \text{ mcg/minute} \times 1 \text{ ml}$$

$$X = \frac{200 \text{ mg}}{500 \text{ ml}}$$

$$X = 0.4 \text{ mg/ml}$$

Dosage drills

Test your math skills with this drill.

> Be sure to show
> how you arrive at
> your answer.

An infusion of norepinephrine (Levophed) containing 4 mg in 250 ml of D₅W is running at 30 ml/hr. How many micrograms of norepinephrine are infusing each minute?

Your answer: _____

Strikeout

Strike out the incorrect equation in the calculation sequence for this problem.

> Congratulations!
> You're finished!

The prescriber orders an I.V. infusion of dobutamine at 7 mcg/kg/minute for a 220-lb patient. The label tells you to check the package insert, which states to dilute 250 mg of the drug in 50 ml of D₅W. Because the drug vial contains 20 ml of solution, the total to be infused is 70 ml (50 ml of D₅W + 20 ml of solution). How many micrograms of the drug the patient should receive each minute?

1. $\dfrac{220 \text{ lb}}{X} = \dfrac{2.2 \text{ lb}}{1 \text{ kg}}$

2. $X \times 2.2 \text{ lb} = 1 \text{ kg} \times 70 \text{ ml}$

3. $\dfrac{X \times \cancel{2.2 \text{ lb}}}{\cancel{2.2 \text{ lb}}} = \dfrac{1 \text{ kg} \times 200 \cancel{\text{ lb}}}{2.2 \cancel{\text{ lb}}}$

4. $X = \dfrac{220}{2.2}$

5. $X = 100 \text{ kg}$

6. $\dfrac{100 \text{ kg}}{X} = \dfrac{1 \text{ kg}}{7 \text{ mcg/minute}}$

7. $X \times 1 \text{ kg} = 7 \text{ mcg/minute} \times 100 \text{ kg}$

8. $\dfrac{X \times \cancel{1 \text{ kg}}}{\cancel{1 \text{ kg}}} = \dfrac{7 \text{ mcg/minute} \times 100 \cancel{\text{ kg}}}{1 \cancel{\text{ kg}}}$

9. $X = 700 \text{ mcg/minute}$

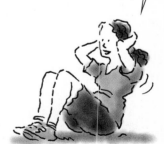

Answers

Chapter 1

■ Page 4

Finish line

1. Numerator, 2. Denominator, 3. Numerator, 4. Denominator

Match point

1. A or C, 2. B, 3. A or C, 4. D

■ Page 5

Hit or miss

1. False. You can manipulate fractions by finding a common denominator.
2. True.
3. True.
4. False. The fraction $3/10$ is already at its lowest terms because 3 and 10 have no common divisor.
5. True.

Finish line

1. $1/4$, 2. $1/8$, 3. $1/16$

■ Page 6

Finish line

1. Hundreds, 2. Tens, 3. Ones, 4. Tenths, 5. Hundredths, 6. Thousandths, 7. Ten thousandths

Strikeout

1. ~~5.34~~. This should be 5.35.
4. ~~7.33~~. This should be 7.32.
5. ~~15.02~~. This should be 15.01.

■ Page 7

Batter's box

1. C, 2. A, 3. B

Starting lineup

Take $1/3$
Divide 1 by 3
Take 0.333
Round to 0.33

■ Page 8

Match point

1. B, 2. C, 3. A

You make the call

Answer: 3 :10 or $3/10$

■ Page 9

Hit or miss

Answer: False. It would take 12 nurses to lift 24 lbs of medical supplies to do this.

Strikeout

$$\frac{\text{~~150 bedpans~~}}{\text{~~1 floor~~}} = \frac{\text{~~325 bedpans~~}}{\text{~~3 floor~~}}$$

The numerator to the right of the equals sign should have been multiplied by 3 to equal 450 bedpans.

Page 10

mble gym

ver: X factor

tter's box

C, 2. A, 3. B

Page 11

arting lineup

rt one

| Multiply the numerators. |
| Multiply the denominators. |
| Restate the equation. |
| Reduce the fraction. |
| nvert the equation to decimal form. |

rt two

| $X = \frac{1}{5} \times \frac{3}{9}$ |
| $1 \times 3 = 3$ |
| $5 \times 9 = 45$ |
| $X = \frac{1 \times 3}{5 \times 9} = \frac{3}{45}$ |
| $X = \frac{3}{3} \div \frac{4}{45} = \frac{1}{15}$ |
| $= \frac{1}{15} = 1 \div 15 = 0.07$ |

Page 12

tter's box

D, 2. C, 3. A, 4. E, 5. B

■ Page 13

You make the call

Answer: Example 1 contains the correct answer.

Strikeout

1. 0.25
2. 1.31
3. 0.13. Because $\frac{2}{15}$ is the correct answer in the previous game, its decimal form, 0.13, is the correct answer here. This form is the result of dividing the fraction's numerator (2) by its denominator (15).
4. 0.19
5. 0.46

■ Page 14

Cross-training

■ Page 15

Starting lineup

| $X = \frac{150}{600} \times \frac{3}{1}$ |
| $X = \frac{150 \times 3}{600 \times 1}$ |
| $X = \frac{450}{600}$ |
| $X = \frac{3}{4} = 3 \div 4 = 0.75$ |

Match point

1. D, 2. B, 3. A, 4. E, 5. C

■ Page 16

Batter's box

1. D, 2. A, 3. G, 4. E, 5. C, 6. H, 7. F, 8. B

Starting lineup

$$X = \frac{25}{12} \times \frac{0.5}{1}$$

$$25 \times 0.5 = 12.5$$

$$12 \times 1 = 12$$

$$X = \frac{25 \times 0.5}{12 \times 1} = \frac{12.5}{12}$$

$$X = \frac{12.5}{12} = 12.5 \div 12 = 1.04$$

■ Page 17

Match point

1. C, 2. A, 3. E, 4. D, 5. B

Hit or miss

Answer: False. The calculation should read as follows:

$$X = \frac{0.44}{0.12 \times 0.5}$$

$$X = \frac{44}{12} \times 0.5$$

$$X = \frac{44}{12} \times \frac{0.5}{1}$$

$$44 \times 0.5 = 22$$

$$12 \times 1 = 12$$

$$X = \frac{44 \times 0.5}{12 \times 1} = \frac{22}{12} = 1.83$$

■ Page 18

Finish line

1. Extreme, 2. Mean, 3. Mean, 4. Extreme

Batter's box

1. F, 2. C, 3. H, 4. B, 5. D, 6. E or G, 7. A, 8. E or G

■ Page 19

Jumble gym

Answer: Extremes

Train your brain

Answer: In a proportion, you can solve for any of four unknow parts.

■ Page 20

Starting lineup

$$20 \times 50 = X \times 10$$

$$1000 = 10X$$

$$\frac{1000}{10} = \frac{10X}{10}$$

$$1000 \div 10 = X$$

$$X = 100$$

$$100 : 20 :: 50 : 10$$

Hit or miss

Answer: True.

■ Page 21

Finish line

1. $\frac{72}{36} = \frac{36X}{36}$
2. $500 \div 20 = X$
3. $X = 10$
4. $X \times 2 = 8 \times 16$

■ Page 22

Multiple reps

Answer: 0.5 ml. Solve by substituting X for the amount of solu needed to administer 0.125 mg of the drug and then set up a proportion with ratios or fractions.

Page 23

tch point

rt one
, 2. A, 3. F, 4. C, 5. B, 6. D

rt two
, 2. B, 3. A, 4. C

Page 24

ish line
0, 2. 90, 3. 90, 4. 30

tter's box
, 2. B, 3. A or C, 4. D, 5. A or C

Page 25

tter's box
, 2. E, 3. A, 4. D, 5. B, 6. F

nble gym
equipment, 2. jumps, 3. **vault**, 4. physique,
er: Equivalents

Page 26

tch point
, 2. A, 3. D, 4. C, 5. H, 6. G, 7. E, 8. F

rikeout
1. 30 ml
2. 30 ml
3. 30 ml
4. There is no cure for this one.

unce is equal to 30 ml.

■ Page 27

Hit or miss
1. True.
2. True.
3. True.
4. False. 64 oz is equal to 1.8 kg.
5. True.

Strikeout
1. 480 oz
2. 320 oz
3. 340 oz
4. 400 oz

Because 1 lb equals 16 oz, 20 lb is the same as 16 oz multiplied
20 times, or 320 oz.

■ Page 28

Match point
Step 1: D, Step 2: F, Step 3: B, Step 4: E, Step 5: A,
Step 6: C

Starting lineup

150 mg

X tsp

1 tsp = 5 ml, 25 mg = 1 ml

$$\frac{1 \text{ tsp}}{5 \text{ ml}} \times \frac{1 \text{ ml}}{25 \text{ mg}} \times \frac{150 \text{ mg}}{1}$$

$$\frac{1 \text{ tsp}}{5 \text{ ml}} \times \frac{1 \text{ ml}}{25 \text{ mg}} \times \frac{150 \text{ mg}}{1}$$

$$1 \text{ tsp} \times 1 \times \frac{150}{5} \times 25 \times 1 =$$
$$\frac{150 \text{ tsp}}{125} = 1.2 \text{ tsp of the suspension}$$

■ **Page 29**

Cross-training

	C			X	F	A	C	T	O	R
	O						R			
	N						O			
	V						S			
	E	X	T	R	E	M	E	S		
	R						M	E	A	N	S
	T						U			
							L		G	
M	I	L	L	I	M	E	T	E	R	
		I					I		A	
		T					P		M	
		E					L			
		R					Y			

■ Chapter 2

■ **Page 34**

Cross-training

			M					
	L		E					
	I		T		D	R	U	G
	T		E					G
M	E	T	R	I	C			R
	R			I		U		A
		C	O	M	M	O	N		M
				A		I		
				L		T		
				S				

■ **Page 35**

Gear up!

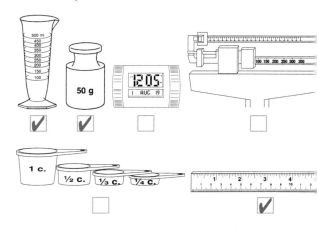

Match point

1. E, 2. G, 3. A, 4. F, 5. B, 6. H, 7. C, 8. I, 9. D

■ **Page 36**

Match point

1. D, 2. B, 3. I, 4. G, 5. C, 6. E, 7. H, 8. F, 9. A

Batter's box

1. B, 2. A, 3. C, 4. A, 5. B, 6. C, 7. B, 8. A

■ **Page 37**

Train your brain

Answer: A cubic centimeter and a milliliter are equal and may used interchangeably.

Hit or miss

1. False. To convert a smaller unit to a larger unit, move the decimal point to the left.
2. True.

age 38

ter's box

ids		Solids	
= $\dfrac{G}{1}$		$\dfrac{E}{6}$ = 1 mg	
) ml = 1 L		1,000 mg = 1 g	
$\dfrac{C}{2}$ = 1 L		100 cg = $\dfrac{B}{7}$	
= $\dfrac{J}{3}$		10 dg = 1 g	
= 1 dkl		10 g = $\dfrac{F}{8}$	
. = $\dfrac{A}{4}$		100 g = $\dfrac{H}{9}$	
$\dfrac{I}{5}$ = 1 kl		$\dfrac{D}{10}$ = 1 kg	

ikeout

3 m
90 m
,000 m
3,000 m

se 1 km equals 1,000 meters, 3 km is equal to 1,000 meters
ied by 3, or 3,000 meters.

age 39

or miss

alse. This works out to 30 g.
rue.

tiple reps

er: 2,013 g. Solve by adding 2,000 g (the equivalent of
3 g (the equivalent of 3,000 mg) and 10 g.

age 40

rting lineup

$$\frac{X}{300,000 \text{ units}} = \frac{1 \text{ ml}}{1,000,000 \text{ units}}$$

$$X \times 1,000,000 \text{ units} = 1 \text{ ml} \times 300,000 \text{ units}$$

$$\frac{1,000,000 \text{ units}}{1,000,000 \text{ units}} = 1\text{ml} \times \frac{300,000 \text{ units}}{1,000,000 \text{ units}}$$

$$X = 0.3 \text{ ml}$$

■ **Page 41**

Finish line

1. 50 ml
2. 20 mEq
3. 20 ml

Jumble gym

1. **units**, 2. **conversion**, 3. international **units**

Answer: Insulin

■ **Page 42**

Hit or miss

Answer: False. This is the drug manufacturer's responsibility.

Finish line

Liquids		
Household	**Apothecaries'**	**Metric**
1 drop (gtt)	1 minim (m)	$\dfrac{0.06 \text{ milliliter (ml)}}{1}$
15 to 16 gtt	15 to 16 m	$\dfrac{1 \text{ ml}}{2}$
$\dfrac{1 \text{ teaspoon (tsp)}}{3}$	1 fluidram	5 ml
1 tablespoon (tbs)	$\dfrac{1/2 \text{ fluid ounce (oz)}}{4}$	15 ml
$\dfrac{2 \text{ tbs}}{5}$	1 fluid oz	30 ml
1 cup	$\dfrac{8 \text{ fluid oz}}{6}$	240 ml
1 pint (pt)	16 fluid oz	$\dfrac{480 \text{ ml}}{7}$
1 quart (qt)	$\dfrac{32 \text{ fluid oz}}{8}$	960 ml
1 gallon (gal)	128 fluid oz	$\dfrac{3,840 \text{ ml}}{9}$

Solids		
Avoirdupois	**Apothecaries'**	**Metric**
1 grain (gr)	1 gr	$\dfrac{0.06 \text{ (g)}}{10}$
1 gr	1 gr	$\dfrac{60 \text{ milligrams (mg)}}{11}$
15.4 gr	$\dfrac{15 \text{ gr}}{12}$	1 g
1 oz	$\dfrac{480 \text{ gr}}{13}$	28.35 g
$\dfrac{1 \text{ pound (lb)}}{14}$	1.33 lb	454 g
2.2 lb	$\dfrac{2.7 \text{ lb}}{15}$	1 kilogram (kg)

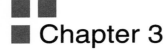

Chapter 3

■ Page 46

Match point

1. D, 2. C, 3. A, 4. B, 5. F, 6. E

Strikeout

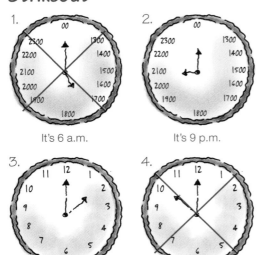

1.
It's 6 a.m.

2.
It's 9 p.m.

3.
It's 0200 hours.

4.
It's 1300 hours.

■ Page 47

Hit or miss

1. False. This abbreviation is no longer considered acceptable.
2. True.
3. False. "Liter" is abbreviated as "L," using upper case.
4. True.
5. False. "DS" is the abbreviation for "double strength."
6. False. "Long-acting" is abbreviated as "la," using lower case.
7. False. These abbreviations are no longer considered acceptable.
8. True.
9. True.
10. True.

Finish line

1. Give 500 mg of Glucophage by mouth twice a day before meals.
2. Begin giving 75 mg of clopidogrel by mouth daily.
3. Increase Demerol to 25 mg intravenously every 4 hours.
4. Give 10 mg of lisinopril by mouth every 8 hours, withhold the drug if the systolic blood pressure falls below 90 mm Hg.
5. Discontinue intravenous famotidine.
6. Give 12.5 to 25 mg of temazepam by mouth at bedtime as needed for sleeplessness.

■ Page 48

Jumble gym

1. date, 2. name, 3. strength, 4. form, 5. route, 6. site, 7. schedule, 8. signature

Answer: Document

Strikeout

1. If a drug order seems questionable, only ask the pharma to check it. If a drug order seems questionable, you shou use all available resources to check it, including the practitioner, the pharmacist, your colleagues, and a drug handbook.
4. It's ok to administer a drug from a vial without a label. Yo should never administer a drug that's improperly labeled missing a label or that you personally didn't draw from a

■ Page 49

Batter's box

1. C, 2. B, 3. D, 4. E, 5. G, 6. F, 7. A

Hit or miss

1. True.
2. True.
3. False. These machines do dispense controlled substance
4. False. Your username and password serve as your signa
5. True.
6. False. If you have to discard any of the dose, have anoth nurse verify the amount discarded and ask her to sign th note as well.
7. True.

■ Page 50

Cross-training

								¹D		
					²N			I		
					A			S		
			³T		M			C		
			H	⁴R	E	C	O	R	D	
⁵F			I					I	N	
⁶A	P	P	R	O	P	R	I	A	T	E
X			T					I		
I			Y					N		
N								U		
G		⁷S	E	Q	U	E	N	C	E	
								D		

age 51

sh line

goxin, furosemide, and famotidine, 2. heparin sodium,
the stop date for glyburide is 9/20, so the nurse shouldn't
ster this drug on 9/21. The practitioner must reevaluate the
4. oral (P.O. route), 5. Yes, the patient is allergic to aspirin.
arin sodium, 7. No, the nurse should mark this as omitted
o state the reason for the omission in the patient's progress
because the MAR provides no space for this information.
they should also document the administration site because
dine is an I.V. drug. 9. When a patient doesn't receive
ation because fasting is required, the nurse should write an
he appropriate blocks and initial them. She should also note
ission and its reason in the patient's progress notes.

age 52

ter's box

t 1: Types of errors

E, B, 2. A, 3. H, 4. I, 5. G, 6. F, 7. C

t 2: Causes

2. B, 3. H, 4. A, 5. G, 6. F, 7. E, 8. C

age 53

ch point

, 2. K, 3. A, 4. C, 5. E, 6. D, 7. B, 8. O, 9. M, 10. H,
, 12. J, 13. L, 14. I, 15. F

age 54

ter's box

, 2. D, 3. E, 4. A, 5. B

or miss

er: True.

age 55

sh line

arbidopa/levodopa, 2. Benztropine, 3. No, it expires on
4. Oral, 5. Yes, aspirin. 6. When a patient doesn't receive
ation because fasting is required, the nurse should write an
he appropriate blocks and initial them. The nurse should also
is omission and its reason in the patient's progress notes.

■ Page 56

Jumble gym

1. identification, 2. first, 3. anyone, 4. bracelet, 5. Replace

Strikeout

2. ~~How medications are listed on the medication administration record~~. It isn't necessary to convey this information to the patient.
4. ~~When patients should discontinue medications before checking with a practitioner~~. Patients should always check with a practitioner before discontinuing medications.

■ Page 57

Starting lineup

Verify the patient's full name.
Check to see if he's wearing allergy identification.
Look for allergy medication on the front of the chart or on the medication record.
Double check the allergy information against the chart.
Ask the patient directly about allergies, even if he's in distress.

Finish line

1. Administer 5 mg of Compazine by intramuscular injection every 6 hours, as needed, for nausea or vomiting. 2. Administer 0.25 mg of digoxin by mouth daily, hold for apical pulse rate less than 60 beats/minute. 3. Immediately administer 50 mg of lidocaine by intravenous bolus infusion at a rate of 25 mg/minute; if necessary, repeat the dose after 8 to 10 minutes, one time only. 4. Administer 20 mg of nifedipine sublingually every 8 hours. 5. Administer 25 mg of hydroxyzine by intramuscular injection every 4 hours, as needed, for anxiety.

■ Page 58

Batter's box

1. C, 2. A, 3. D, 4. B

Hit or miss

1. True.
2. True.
3. False. These patients shouldn't receive sulfonylurea hypoglycemic agents.

■ Page 59
Starting lineup

> The practitioner must choose the right medication for the patient, then write the order correctly and legibly.

> The pharmacist must interpret the order, determine whether it's complete, and prepare the drug using precise measurements.

> The nurse must evaluate whether the medication is appropriate for the patient, then administer it correctly according to facility guidelines.

Jumble gym
1. compound, 2. medication, 3. error, 4. team, 5. double-check, 6. drugs

Answer: Pharmacist

■ Page 60
Strikeout
5. ~~Choosing the right medication for the patient~~. This is the practitioner's responsibility.

Hit or miss
Answer: True.

■ Page 61
Batter's box
1. B, 2. C, 3. H, 4. D, 5. F, 6. E, 7. G, 8. A

Match point
1. B, 2. C, 3. D, 4. E, 5. F, 6. A

■ Page 62
Hit or miss
1. False. Verbal orders to administer a drug are typically given during emergencies when there's no time to write out an order.
2. True.
3. False. This is necessary.
4. True.
5. True.

Batter's box
1. C, 2. E, 3. A, 4. D, 5. B

■ Page 63
Batter's box
1. E, 2. G, 3. B, 4. H, 5. C, 6. A, 7. F, 8. D

Jumble gym
1. responsibility, 2. errors, 3. minimize, 4. drug, 5. administration

Answer: Stress

■ Page 64
Batter's box
1. C, 2. B, 3. E, 4. A, 5. F, 6. D

■ Page 65
Strikeout
2. ~~Administering the drug is against your religious or ethical beliefs.~~
4. ~~You think that the prescribed dosage is too low.~~
5. ~~You think that the patient would be better helped by a different drug instead.~~

Starting lineup

> Notify the practitioner.

> Consult the pharmacist.

> Follow your facility's policy for documenting drug errors.

> Consider reporting the error to the United States Pharmacop[

Chapter 4

age 69

or miss

alse. Drugs that are administered orally are usually in tablet,
apsule, or liquid form.
rue.
alse. This ability is essential to nursing.
rue.
rue.
alse. If the drug has two names, the generic name typically
ppears in lowercase, not uppercase, print.
rue.

sh line

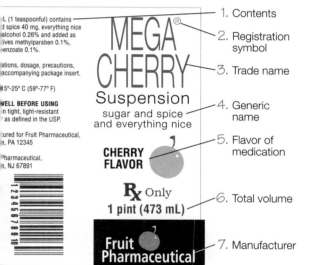

L (1 teaspoonful) contains
d spice 40 mg, everything nice
alcohol 0.26% and added as
ives methylparaben 0.1%,
enzoate 0.1%.

ations, dosage, precautions,
accompanying package insert.

5°-25° C (59°-77° F)

NELL BEFORE USING
n tight, light-resistant
as defined in the USP.

tured for Fruit Pharmaceutical,
e, PA 12345

Pharmaceutical,
e, NJ 67891

MEGA® CHERRY
Suspension
sugar and spice
and everything nice

CHERRY FLAVOR

Rx Only
1 pint (473 mL)

Fruit Pharmaceutical

1. Contents
2. Registration symbol
3. Trade name
4. Generic name
5. Flavor of medication
6. Total volume
7. Manufacturer

■ Page 70

Finish line

1. Administer 325 mg of ferrous sulfate by mouth three times a
day before meals. 2. Administer 10 mg of Procardia by mouth
three times a day and as needed for systolic blood pressure
greater than 180 mm Hg. 3. Administer four 1-gram doses of
oxacillin by piggyback intravenous infusion, 6 hours apart.
4. Administer 5% dextrose in Ringer's lactate solution by
intravenous infusion at a rate of 100 ml/hour. 5. Place 2 drops of
0.5% Chloroptic solution in the right eye every 6 hours.

Dosage drills

1,000 mg : 1 g :: 1,500 mg : X g

1,000 mg $\times$ X g = 1 g $\times$ 1,500 mg

$1,000X = 1,500$

$X = \dfrac{1,500}{1,000}$

$X = 1.5$ g

0.5 g : 1 tab :: 1.5 g : X tab

0.5 g $\times$ X = 1 $\times$ 1.5 g

$0.5 X = 1.5$

$X = \dfrac{1.5}{0.5}$

$X = 3$ tablets

■ Page 71

Batter's box

1. C, 2. B, 3. A, 4. F, 5. E, 6. G, 7. D

Out of bounds

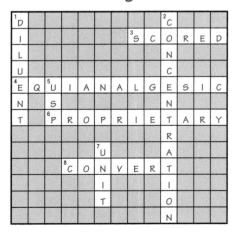

■ Page 72

Cross-training

¹D						²C					
I				³S	C	O	R	E	D		
L						N					
U						C					
⁴E	⁵Q	U	I	A	N	A	L	G	E	S	I	C
N	S					N					
T		⁶P	R	O	P	R	I	E	T	A	R	Y
						R					
			⁷U			A					
		⁸C	O	N	V	E	R	T			
			I			T					
			T			I					
						O					
						N					

■ Page 73

Starting lineup

> Open the patient's medication drawer, find the drug labeled metoclopramide (Reglan) 10 mg, and note that it's in oral tablet form.

> Place the labeled drug next to the transcribed order on the administration record and carefully compare each part of the label to the order.

> If the drug is supplied in bulk or in a stock bottle, transfer one tablet from the supply to a medication contain pouring from the supply to the lid and then into a containe without handling the tablet.

> Before returning the supply to the drawer or shelf, once ag compare the label to the order on the administration recor and note whether this is the right administration time.

> Go to the patient's bedside, check his identification bracel and do your third drug check, comparing the label to the or and checking the administration time again. Then give the d

> If the drug comes in a unit-dose packet, don't remove it fro the packet until you're at the patient's bedside and ready administer it. Then do your third drug check. Remove the d from the packet and give it to the patient, using the packet la for comparison when recording your administration informat

■ Page 74

Dosage drills

500 mg : 5 ml : : 200 mg : X ml

500 mg $\times$ X ml = 5 ml $\times$ 200 mg

$500X = 1,000$

$X = \dfrac{1,000}{500}$

$X = 2$ ml

Hit or miss

1. True.
2. True.
3. False. The pharmacist performs this task.
4. False. Many, but not all, facilities use the unit-dose syster

Page 75

atter's box

. D, 2. F, 3. A, 4. E, 5. C, 6. B

osage drills

g : 15 ml : : 25 g : X ml

g × X ml = 15 ml × 25 g

X = 375

$\frac{375}{10}$

37.5 ml

Page 76

arting lineup

| 0.025 mg : 1 tablet : : 0.05 mg : X |

| tablet × 0.05 mg = 0.025 mg × X |

| $\frac{\text{tablet} \times 0.05 \text{ mg}}{0.025 \text{ mg}} = \frac{0.025 \text{ mg} \times X}{0.025 \text{ mg}}$ |

mble gym

measure, 2. decimals, 3. calculator, 4. solve, 5. means,
extremes

ver: Double-check

Page 77

sage drills

g : 1 tab : : 30 : X

g × X tab = 1 tab × 30 mg

= 30

30
.5

tablets

or miss

alse. Most tablets, capsules, and similar dose forms are
vailable in only a few strengths.
ue.
ue.
alse. In these cases, you should substitute a commercially
vailable solution or suspension or have one prepared by the
harmacist.
ue.
ue.

■ Page 78

Hit or miss

Answer: True.

Batter's box

1. D, 2. G, 3. A, 4. H, 5. E, 6. C, 7. F, 8. B

■ Page 79

Jumble gym

Answer: Proportions

Dosage drills

0.05 mg : 1 ml : : 0.125 mg : X ml

0.05 mg × X ml = 0.125 mg × 1 ml

$\frac{0.05 \text{ mg} \times X \text{ ml}}{0.05 \text{ mg}} = \frac{0.125 \text{ mg} \times 1 \text{ ml}}{0.05 \text{ mg}}$

$X = \frac{0.125}{0.05}$

X = 2.5 ml

■ Page 80

Dosage drills

40 mg : 1 tab : : 100 mg : X tab

40 mg × X tab = 100 mg × 1 tab

$\frac{40 \text{ mg} \times X \text{ tab}}{40 \text{ mg}} = \frac{100 \text{ mg} \times 1 \text{ tab}}{40 \text{ mg}}$

$X = \frac{100}{40}$

X = 2.5 tablets

Starting lineup

| $\frac{5 \text{ ml}}{250 \text{ mg}}$ |

| $\frac{X}{500 \text{ mg}}$ |

| $\frac{X}{500 \text{ mg}} = \frac{5 \text{ ml}}{250 \text{ mg}}$ |

| $X \times 250 \text{ mg} = 5 \text{ ml} \times 500 \text{ mg}$ |

| $\frac{X \times 250 \text{ mg}}{250 \text{ mg}} = \frac{5 \text{ ml} \times 500 \text{ mg}}{250 \text{ mg}}$ |

| $X = \frac{2,500 \text{ ml}}{250}$ |

| X = 10 ml |

■ Page 81

Batter's box

1. C, 2. B, 3. D, 4. E, 5. A

Dosage drills

40 mEq : 30 ml : : X mEq : 15 ml

40 mEq $\times$ 15 ml = 30 ml $\times$ X mEq

$$\frac{40 \text{ mEq} \times 15 \text{ ml}}{30 \text{ ml}} = \frac{30 \text{ ml} \times X \text{ mEq}}{30 \text{ ml}}$$

$$\frac{600}{30} = X$$

X = 20 mEq

■ Page 82

Dosage drills

200 mg : 1 tab : : 600 mg : X tab

200 mg $\times$ X tab = 1 tab $\times$ 600 mg

$$\frac{200 \text{ mg} \times X \text{ tab}}{200 \text{ mg}} = \frac{1 \text{ tab} \times 600 \text{ mg}}{200 \text{ mg}}$$

$$X = \frac{600}{200}$$

X = 3 tablets

Hit or miss

1. True.
2. False. You should hold the cup at eye level, not above, for accuracy.
3. False. You should hold the solution with the medication label turned toward, not away from, the palm of your hand for this purpose.
4. True.
5. False. Standard droppers can and should be used for this purpose.
6. True.
7. True.

■ Page 83

Dosage drills

4 mg : 1 ml : : 10 mg : X ml

4 mg $\times$ X ml = 10 mg $\times$ 1 ml

$4X$ = 10

$$X = \frac{10}{4}$$

X = 2.5 ml

■ Page 84

Match point

1. B, 2. H, 3. A, 4. E, 5. F, 6. I, 7. D, 8. G, 9. C

Dosage drills

500,000 units : 5 ml : : 300,000 units : X ml

500,000 units $\times$ X ml = 5 ml $\times$ 300,000 units

$$\frac{500,000 \text{ units} \times X \text{ ml}}{500,000 \text{ units}} = \frac{5 \text{ ml} \times 300,000 \text{ units}}{500,000 \text{ units}}$$

$$X = \frac{1,500,000}{500,000}$$

X = 3 ml

■ Page 85

Dosage drills

1 g : 1,000 mg : : 2 g : X mg

1 g $\times$ X mg = 1,000 mg $\times$ 2 g

X = 2,000 mg

500 mg : 5 ml : : 2,000 mg : X ml

500 $\times$ X = 5 $\times$ 2,000

500X = 10,000

X = 20 ml

Batter's box

1. B, 2. C, 3. A

CHAPTER 4

219

Page 86

tarting lineup

Convert the milliliters to tablespoons by using a conversion table.
Set up the first fraction with the amount desired over the amount you have.
et up the second fraction with the unknown amount desired (*X*) in the appropriate position.
Put the fractions into a proportion.
Cross-multiply the fractions.
Solve for *X* by dividing each side of the equation by 30 mg and canceling units that appear in both the numerator and denominator.

sage drills

ng : 1 tablet : : 50 mg : *X* tablets

let × 50 mg = 20 mg × *X* tablets

= 50

50
20

2.5 tablets

Page 87

tch point

3, 2. C, 3. D, 4. A, 5. E

sage drills

ng : 5 ml : : 500 mg : *X* ml

g × *X* ml = 5 ml × 500 mg

$$\frac{g \times X \, ml}{5 \, mg} = \frac{5 \, ml \times 500 \, mg}{125 \, mg}$$

,500
125

) ml

■ Page 88

Cross-training

		¹A							
	²D	E	R	M	A	L			
		M						³P	
		I						A	
	⁴E	N	E	M	A	S		T	
		I							
⁵N	A	S	O	G	A	S	T	⁶R	I	C
		T					E	C	H
⁷D	E	R	M	I	S			C	
		A						T	
		T			⁸T	R	A	D	E
		I						L	
⁹P	O	W	D	E	R	S			
		N							

■ Page 89

Finish line

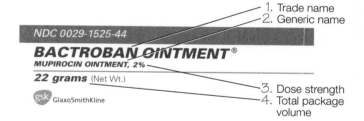

1. Trade name
2. Generic name
3. Dose strength
4. Total package volume

Dosage drills

X mg : 20 gr : : 60 mg : 1 gr

X mg × 1 gr = 20 gr × 60 mg

X = 1,200 mg

X capsules : 1,200 mg : : 1 capsule : 300 mg

300 mg × *X* capsules = 1,200 mg × 1 capsule

300 *X* = 1,200

$$X = \frac{1,200}{300}$$

X = 4 capsules

■ Page 90
Dosage drills

325 mg : 5 ml : : 650 mg : X ml

325 mg $\times$ X ml = 650 mg $\times$ 5 ml

$325X = 3,250$

$X = \frac{3,250}{325}$

$X = 10$ ml

5 ml : 1 teaspoon : : 10 ml : X teaspoons

5 ml $\times$ X teaspoons = 1 teaspoon $\times$ 10 ml

$5X = 10$

$X = \frac{10}{5}$

$X = 2$ teaspoons

Hit or miss

1. True.
2. False. Today, topical drugs are also used for their systemic effects.
3. False. These drugs are absorbed into the circulation.
4. True.
5. True.
6. False. Patches are used precisely because they maintain consistent blood levels of a drug.
7. True.
8. False. Reversing these effects can be difficult because the drug takes so long to be metabolized.

■ Page 91
Dosage drills

1 mg : 1,000 mcg : 0.25 mg : X mcg

1 mg $\times$ X mcg = 1,000 mcg $\times$ 0.25 mg

$X = 250$ mcg

250 mcg : X tablets : 125 mcg : 1 tablet

250 mcg $\times$ 1 tablet = 125 mcg $\times$ X tablets

$250 = 125X$

$X = \frac{250}{125}$

$X = 2$ tablets

Batter's box

1. C, 2. A, 3. B, 4. E, 5. D

■ Page 92
Match point

1. F, 2. D, 3. B, 4. A, 5. E, 6. C

Strikeout

3. ~~Habitrol, Nicoderm, Nicotrol, and ProStep should be used without other therapy.~~ These drugs should be used as adjuncts to behavioral therapy.
4. ~~Transdermal fentanyl is administered to treat hypertension.~~ This drug is used to treat severe chronic pain.
7. ~~The clonidine patch is used to treat hypotension.~~ This patch used to treat hypertension, not hypotension.

■ Page 93
Jumble gym

1. absorption, 2. apply, 3. blood, 4. local, 5. onset, 6. tolerance, 7. transdermal

Answer: Displaced

Dosage drills

1 supp : 325 mg

X supp : 650 mg

1 supp : 325 mg : : X supp : 650 mg

325 mg $\times$ X supp = 650 mg $\times$ 1 supp

$\frac{325\ \text{mg} \times X\ \text{supp}}{325\ \text{mg}} = \frac{650\ \text{mg} \times 1\ \text{supp}}{325\ \text{mg}}$

$X = 2$ suppositories

■ Page 94
Dosage drills

800 mg : X tablets : : 400 mg : 1 tablet

800 mg $\times$ 1 tablet = 400 mg $\times$ X tablets

$800 = 400X$

$X = \frac{800}{400}$

$X = 2$ tablets

Batter's box

1. D, A, 2. C, 3. B

Page 95

osage drills

mg : X supp :: 5 mg : 1 supp

mg × 1 supp = 5 mg × X supp

= 5X

= $\frac{10}{5}$

= 2 suppositories

atch point

. B, 2. A, 3. C, 4. A, 5. A, 6. A

Page 96

t or miss

False. Patches are changed at regular intervals to ensure that the patient receives the correct dose.
False. The old patch should be removed before the new patch is applied.
False. When applying ointment from a tube, use a paper ruler applicator to measure the correct dose.

tter's box

F, 2. G, 3. E, 4. B, 5. C, 6. A, 7. D

Page 97

sage drills

ng : 1 tab :: 1,000 mg : X tab

ng × X tab = 1 tab × 1,000 mg

$\frac{ng \times X\,tab}{00\,mg} = \frac{1\,tab \times 1,000\,mg}{500\,mg}$

$\frac{,000}{500}$

tablets

sh line

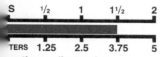

NITRO-BID®
troglycerin Ointment USP, 2%)

the applicator that
measures the dose
E. FOUGERA & CO.
a division of Altana Inc.
MELVILLE, NEW YORK 11747

■ Page 98

Hit or miss

1. True.
2. True.
3. False. The practitioner usually, not rarely, prescribes drugs in the dose provided by one suppository, but occasionally you may need to insert two suppositories.

Starting lineup

Set up the first fraction with the known suppository dose.
Set up the second fraction with the desired dose and the unknown number of suppositories.
Put the first and second fractions into a proportion.
Cross-multiply the fractions.
Solve for X by dividing each side of the equation by 60 mg and canceling units that appear in both the numerator and denominator.

■ Page 99

Dosage drills

100 mg : 15 ml :: 400 mg : X ml

100 mg × X ml = 15 mg × 400 mg

$\frac{100\,mg \times X\,ml}{100\,mg} = \frac{15\,mg \times 400\,mg}{100\,mg}$

$X = \frac{6,000}{100}$

$X = 60$ ml

Hit or miss

Answer: False. You would give ½.

■ Page 100

Match point

1. C, 2. A, 3. B

Dosage drills

500 mg : 1 tab :: 750 mg : X tab

500 mg × X tab = 1 tab × 750 mg

$\frac{500\,mg \times X\,tab}{500\,mg} = \frac{1\,tab \times 750\,mg}{500\,mg}$

$X = \frac{750}{500}$

$X = 1.5$ tablets

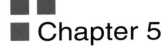 Chapter 5

■ Page 103

Hit or miss

1. True.
2. True.
3. False. Powdered drug forms always require reconstitution.
4. False. You need to perform calculations to determine the amount of liquid medication to inject when using a liquid or powder parenteral drug.

Jumble gym

1. intradermal, 2. subcutaneous, 3. intramuscular

■ Page 104

Batter's box

1. B, 2. A, 3. C, 4. D

Hit or miss

1. True.
2. False. The epidermis is the outermost layer of skin.
3. False. This injection is often used to anesthetize the skin for invasive procedures.
4. True.
5. False. This injection is used to test for histoplasmosis.

■ Page 105

Starting lineup

Clean the skin thoroughly.
Stretch the skin taut with one hand.
Insert the needle quickly at a 10- to 15-degree angle to a depth of about 0.5 cm.
Inject the drug.

Batter's box

1. D, 2. C, 3. E, 4. F, 5. H, 6. G, 7. A, 8. B

■ Page 106

Strikeout

3. ~~The needles used for subQ injections are $3/4''$ to $1''$ long.~~ The needles used for subQ injections are $1/2''$ to $5/8''$ long.
5. ~~The abdomen isn't a subQ injection site.~~ The abdomen is a subQ injection site.

Starting lineup

Choose the injection site.
Clean the skin.
Pinch the patient's skin between your index finger and thumb and insert the needle.
Aspirate for blood to make sure that the needle isn't in a vein (unless injecting insulin or heparin).
Administer the injection.
Massage the site (unless you're giving insulin or heparin).

■ Page 107

Cross-training

```
              1V        2D
        3F E M O R I S
              N         A
        4M    T         M
         A    R    5N E E D L E
         S    A         T
    6M U S C L E        E
                   7V   R
                    O
              8S H A L L O W
                    U
                    M
                    E
```

Page 108

atter's box

1. C, 2. D, 3. F, 4. A, 5. E, 6. B

trikeout

1. ~~Seven basic types of hypodermic syringes are used to measure and administer parenteral drugs.~~ Three, not seven, basic types of hypodermic syringes are used to measure and administer parenteral drugs.

Page 109

t or miss

False. Standard syringes are available in 3, 5, 10, 20, 30, 50, and 60 ml.
True.
False. The dead space holds the fluid that remains in the syringe and needle after the plunger is completely, not partially, depressed.
False. Some syringes, such as insulin syringes, don't have dead space.

rikeout

~~The 5-ml syringe is the most commonly used syringe.~~ The 3-ml syringe is the most commonly used syringe. ~~The large-volume syringes are calibrated in 1- to 5-ml increments.~~ The large-volume syringes are calibrated in 2- to 10-ml increments.

Page 110

ish line

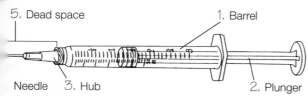

5. Dead space   1. Barrel
Needle   3. Hub   2. Plunger

arting lineup

| Calculate the dose. |
| Use aseptic technique. |
| Draw the drug into the syringe. |
| Pull the plunger back until the top ring of the plunger's black portion aligns with the correct calibration mark. |
| Double-check the dose measurement. |
| Administer the drug. |

■ Page 111

Hit or miss

1. True.
2. False. This dose can be contained in 1 to 3 ml of solution.
3. True.
4. False. Giving the patient this dose in two (not three) injections at two (not three) different sites allows for proper drug absorption.

Batter's box

1. B, 2. E, 3. D, 4. C, 5. A

■ Page 112

Hit or miss

1. True.
2. True.
3. False. Each prefilled cartridge is calibrated in tenths (not hundredths) of a milliliter and has larger (not smaller) marks for half and full milliliters.
4. False. Some cartridges are designed so that a diluent or a second drug can be added when a combined dose is ordered.
5. True.

Strikeout

3. ~~Most manufacturers include the exact amount of a drug in a prefilled syringe.~~ Most manufacturers add a little extra drug to the syringe in case some is wasted when the syringe is purged of air.
4. ~~Prefilled syringes are available in all doses.~~ These syringes aren't available in all doses.
5. ~~You should carefully document the amount of any drug you discard from a prefilled syringe.~~ You should only document this in the case of opioids.

■ Page 113

Finish line

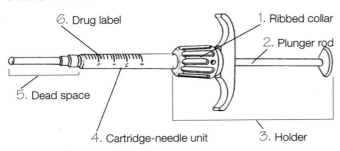

6. Drug label
1. Ribbed collar
2. Plunger rod
5. Dead space
4. Cartridge-needle unit
3. Holder

Starting lineup

Hold the drug chamber in one hand and the syringe and needle in the other.

Flip the protective caps off both ends of the closed-system device.

Insert the drug chamber into the syringe section.

Remove the needle cap and expel air and extra medication.

■ Page 114

Batter's box

1. C, 2. A, 3. B, 4. D, 5. E

Match point

1. D, 2. B, 3. A, 4. E, 5. C

■ Page 115

Starting lineup

$\dfrac{50 \text{ mg}}{1 \text{ ml}}$

$\dfrac{25 \text{ mg}}{X}$

50 mg/1 ml = 25 mg/X

50 mg × X = 25 mg × 1 ml

$\dfrac{\cancel{50 \text{ mg}} \times X}{50 \text{ mg}} = \dfrac{25 \text{ mg} \times 1 \text{ ml}}{50 \text{ mg}}$

$X = \dfrac{25 \text{ ml}}{50}$

$X = 0.5$ ml

■ Page 116

Match point

1. E, 2. A, 3. D, 4. B, 5. C

Finish line

1. Total volume of solution
2. Name of drug
3. Dose strength or concentration

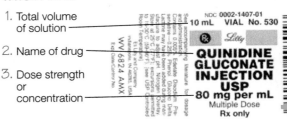

Page 117

tarting lineup

100 mg : 1 ml

120 mg : X

100 mg : 1 ml : : 120 mg : X

1 ml × 120 mg = 100 mg × X

$\dfrac{1 \text{ ml} \times 120 \text{ mg}}{100 \text{ mg}} = \dfrac{100 \text{ mg} \times X}{100 \text{ mg}}$

$X = \dfrac{120 \text{ ml}}{100}$

X = 1.2 ml

Page 118

t or miss

True.
True.
False. A solute is a liquid or solid form of a drug.
True.
False. In this solution, the salt is the solute and the purified
water is the solvent.

tter's box

G, 2. F, 3. B, 4. E, 5. C, 6. A, 7. D

Page 119

tch point

, 2. C, 3. B, 4. A

or miss

alse. This should be grams (not milliliters) solute/100 ml
nished solution.
alse. This should be milliliters (not grams) solute/100 ml
nished solution.
rue.
rue.

■ Page 120

Cross-training

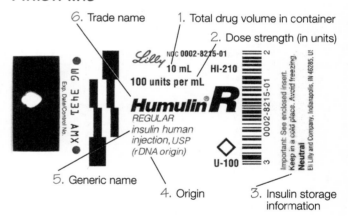

■ Page 121

Finish line

6. Trade name   1. Total drug volume in container
2. Dose strength (in units)

5. Generic name   4. Origin   3. Insulin storage information

Strikeout

2. ~~Type 1 diabetes is also known as *non-insulin-dependent diabetes.*~~ Type 1 diabetes is also known as *insulin-dependent diabetes.*
3. ~~Type 1 diabetes is typically diagnosed after age 30.~~ Type 1 diabetes is typically diagnosed before age 20.
5. ~~The incidence of Type 2 diabetes among children is declining.~~ The incidence of Type 2 diabetes among children is rising, not declining.

■ Page 122

Hit or miss

1. False. Heparin is used in moderate, not large, doses to prevent these diseases.
2. True.
3. True.
4. False. Heparin is available in many concentrations.

Batter's box

1. B, 2. D, 3. K, 4. C, 5. I, 6. H, 7. G, 8. E, 9. F, 10. A, 11. J

■ Page 123

Strikeout

3. ~~Insulin doses are available in three concentrations.~~ Insulin doses are available in two, not three, concentrations.
5. ~~U-500 insulin is called *universal*.~~ U-100 insulin, not U-500 insulin, is called *universal* because it's the most common concentration.

Match point

1. B, 2. C, 3. A

■ Page 124

Hit or miss

1. True.
2. True.
3. False. This type of insulin is considered intermediate acting.
4. False. This type of insulin has an onset of 1 to 2 hours.
5. False. This type of insulin is considered rapid acting.
6. True.
7. True.
8. False. This type of insulin peaks in 10 to 30 hours.
9. True.
10. True.

Batter's box

1. E, 2. A, 3. C, 4. D, 5. B

■ Page 125

Starting lineup

Read the vial labels carefully.

Roll the NPH vial between your palms to mix it thoroughly.

Clean the tops of both vials of insulin with alcohol swabs.

Inject air into the NPH vial equal to the amount of insulin you need to give. Withdraw the needle and syringe, but don't withdraw any NPH insulin.

Inject into the regular insulin vial an amount of air equal to the dose of the regular insulin. Then withdraw the prescribed amount of regular insulin into the syringe.

Clean the top of the NPH vial again. Then insert the needle of the syringe containing the regular insulin into the vial, and withdraw the prescribed amount of NPH insulin.

Mix the insulins in the syringe.

Recheck the drug order.

■ Page 126

Match point

1. C, 2. A, 3. B, 4. E, 5. D

■ Page 127

Finish line

1. No insulin, 2. 2 units regular insulin, 3. 4 units regular insulin, 4. 6 units regular insulin, 5. 8 units regular insulin, 6. N/A, you should call the practitioner for an insulin order.

■ Page 128

Batter's box

1. I, 2. F, 3. C, 4. D, 5. H, 6. E, 7. B, 8. G, 9. A

Page 129

inish line

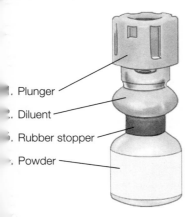

1. Plunger
2. Diluent
3. Rubber stopper
4. Powder

rikeout

~~When a diluent is added to a powder, the fluid volume decreases.~~ When a diluent is added to a powder, the fluid volume increases, not decreases.
~~The label of the powder container calls for more diluent than the total volume of prepared solution.~~ The label of the powder container calls for less, not more, diluent than the total volume of prepared solution.

Page 130

t or miss

False. These vials have two chambers separated by a rubber stopper, not a plunger.
True.
False. When the top of the vial is depressed, the stopper dislodges, allowing the diluent to flow into the lower, not upper, chamber.
True.
True.

rikeout

~~The package inserts that are included with drugs don't usually provide information other than what is on the outer label.~~ Package inserts usually provide more information than what's on the outer label.

■ Page 131

Hit or miss

1. True.
2. False. It's necessary to label this drug with several pieces of information.
3. True.
4. False. The drug should be labeled with the expiration date and dose strength in addition to your initials and the reconstitution date.

Starting lineup

$$\frac{500 \text{ mg}}{20 \text{ ml}}$$

$$\frac{300 \text{ mg}}{X}$$

$$\frac{500 \text{ mg}}{20 \text{ ml}} = \frac{300 \text{ mg}}{X}$$

$$20 \text{ ml} \times 300 \text{ mg} = X \times 500 \text{ mg}$$

$$\frac{20 \text{ ml} \times 300 \text{ mg}}{500 \text{ mg}} = \frac{X \times 500 \text{ mg}}{500 \text{ mg}}$$

$$X = \frac{6000 \text{ ml}}{500}$$

$$X = 12 \text{ ml}$$

■ Page 132

Match point

1. B, 2. A, 3. D, 4. E, 5. C

■ Chapter 6

■ Page 135

Batter's box

1. C, 2. H, 3. E, 4. A, 5. I, 6. B, 7. F, 8. G, 9. D

■ Page 136

Finish line

1. Total volume of I.V. bag, 2. Name and concentration of I.V. fluid, 3. Graduations for measuring

■ Page 137

Batter's box

1. E, 2. C, 3. A, 4. B, 5. D

Hit or miss

1. True.
2. False. This is a relatively slow infusion rate, so you should select microdrip tubing for it.
3. True.

■ Page 138

Strikeout

2. ~~You should use macrodrip tubing for infusions for pediatric patients.~~ You should use microdrip tubing for pediatric infusions to prevent fluid overload.

Match point

1. B, 2. D, 3. A, 4. E, 5. C

■ Page 139

Batter's box

1. B, 2. C, 3. D, 4. A

Starting lineup

Convert 1 hour to 60 minutes to fit the formula.

$$\frac{175\ ml}{60\ minutes}$$

$$X = \frac{175\ \cancel{ml}}{60\ minutes} \times \frac{15\ gtt}{\cancel{ml}}$$

$$X = \frac{175 \times 15\ gtt}{60\ minutes}$$

$$X = \frac{2{,}625\ gtt}{60\ minutes}$$

$$X = \frac{43.75\ gtt}{minute}$$

■ Page 140

Batter's box

1. C, 2. E, 3. A, 4. G, 5. B, 6. F, 7. D

■ Page 141

Hit or miss

1. True.
2. False. This is the number of milliliters of fluid to administer o͏ 1 hour, not 2 hours.
3. True.
4. True.
5. False. You should use the formula of total volume ordered/numbers of hours.

Batter's box

1. C, 2. D, 3. B, 4. A, 5. E

■ Page 142

Match point

1. B, 2. A, 3. D, 4. C

Hit or miss

Answer: True.

■ Page 143

Batter's box

1. B, 2. C, 3. E, 4. A, 5. D

Starting lineup

Determine the flow rate (X) by dividing the number of millilite͏ to be delivered by the number of hours.

Remember the rule: for a set that delivers 15 gtt/ml, divide the flow rate by 4 to determine the drip rate.

Set up an equation to determine the drip rate, which now becomes X, and solve for X. Divide the flow rate by 4.

Page 144

trikeout

3. ~~Computing the time required for infusion of a specified volume of I.V. fluid won't help you perform laboratory tests on time.~~ This will help you perform laboratory tests, such as the chemistry and electrolyte assessments that commonly accompany infusions, on time.

atter's box

1. A, 2. B, 3. E, 4. D, 5. F, 6. C

Page 145

tarting lineup

> Set up the fraction with the volume of the infusion as the numerator and the flow rate as the denominator.

> Solve for X by dividing 1,000 by 50 and canceling units that appear in both the numerator and denominator.

osage drills

: 500 ml = 1 hr : X ml

$\times X$ ml = 500 ml $\times$ 1 hr

$$\frac{\times X \text{ ml}}{2 \text{ hr}} = \frac{500 \text{ ml} \times 1 \text{ hr}}{2 \text{ hr}}$$

$$\frac{500}{2}$$

250 ml/hr

Page 146

t or miss

wer: False. It will be done at 10:00 AM.

tter's box

B, 2. A, 3. D, 4. C, 5. E

■ Page 147

Dosage drills

125 ml : 1 hr : : 1,000 ml : X hr

125 ml $\times$ X hr = 1 hr $\times$ 1,000 ml

$$\frac{125 \text{ ml} \times X \text{ hr}}{125 \text{ ml}} = \frac{1 \text{ hr} \times 1,000 \text{ ml}}{125 \text{ ml}}$$

$$X = \frac{1,000}{125}$$

X = 8 hr

100 ml : 1 hr : : 1,000 ml : X hr

100 ml $\times$ X hr = 1 hr $\times$ 1,000 ml

$$\frac{100 \text{ ml} \times X \text{ hr}}{100 \text{ ml}} = \frac{1 \text{ hr} \times 1,000 \text{ ml}}{100 \text{ ml}}$$

$$X = \frac{1,000}{100}$$

X = 10 hr

8 hours + 10 hours = 18 hours

■ Page 148

Starting lineup

> Infusion time = $\dfrac{500 \text{ ml}}{\left(\dfrac{64 \text{ gtt/minute}}{15 \text{ gtt/minute}}\right) \times 60 \text{ minutes}}$

> $\dfrac{64 \text{ gtt}}{1 \text{ min}} \times \dfrac{1 \text{ ml}}{15 \text{ gtt}} = \dfrac{64 \text{ ml}}{15 \text{ min}} = 4.27 \text{ ml/min}$

> $X = \dfrac{500 \text{ ml}}{\dfrac{4.27 \text{ ml}}{1 \text{ min}} \times \dfrac{60 \text{ min}}{1 \text{ hour}}}$

> $X = \dfrac{500}{4.27 \times 60 \text{ hours}}$

> $X = \dfrac{500}{256.2 \text{ hours}}$

> $X = \dfrac{500}{256 \text{ hours}}$

> X = 1.95 hours

> 1.95 hours $\times$ 60 minutes = 117 minutes

> X = 1 hour 57 minutes

■ Page 149

Hit or miss

Answer: False.

Dosage drills

1400 − 1000 = 4 hours

1 hr: 100 ml : : 4 hr : X ml

1 hr × X ml = 100 ml × 4 hr

$$\frac{\cancel{1 \text{ hr}} \times X \text{ ml}}{1 \text{ hr}} = \frac{100 \text{ ml} \times 4 \cancel{\text{ hr}}}{1 \cancel{\text{ hr}}}$$

X = 100 × 4

X = 400 ml

1 L = 1000 ml

1000 ml − 400 ml = 600 ml remaining

Answer: 600 ml

■ Page 150

Strikeout

1. ~~You can only regulate I.V. flow by using a pump.~~ You can regulate I.V. flow not only by using a pump, you can also regulate it manually or by using a patient-controlled analgesia pump.
2. ~~You can only regulate I.V. flow manually.~~ You can regulate I.V. flow not only manually, you can also regulate it by using a pump or using a patient-controlled analgesia pump.

Batter's box

1. A, 2. D, 3. B, 4. E, 5. C

■ Page 151

Batter's box

1. G, 2. A, 3. D, 4. F, 5. E, 6. B, 7. H, 8. C

Hit or miss

1. False. To time-tape an I.V. bag, place a strip of adhesive tape from the top to the bottom, not from the bottom to the top, of the bag.
2. True.
3. False. You should mark the time at which the solution will be completely infused at the bottom of the tape.
4. True.
5. True.

■ Page 152

Strikeout

3. ~~Currently there are no electronic infusion pumps that have devices which prevent them from pumping fluids into infiltrat sites.~~ These types of pumps do currently exist.
5. ~~Electronic infusion pumps are foolproof.~~ These pumps can make mistakes, they don't eliminate the need for careful calculations and assessment of infusion rates over time.

Batter's box

1. B, 2. A, 3. C, 4. F, 5. E, 6. D

■ Page 153

Hit or miss

1. True.
2. False. The nurse, not the patient, programs this pump.
3. True.
4. False. Blood concentrations of analgesics remain consisten, not inconsistent, throughout the day, which gives the PCA pump an advantage, not a disadvantage, over the traditiona approach.
5. True.

Strikeout

2. ~~Drug dose is programmed on PCA pumps, but administrati frequency is not.~~ Both drug doses and administration frequency are programmed into PCA pumps to prevent the patient from medicating himself too often.
3. ~~If the patient tries to overmedicate himself, the PCA pump machine sounds an alarm.~~ If the patient tries to overmedica himself, the PCA pump ignores the request, it doesn't sour an alarm.

■ Page 154

Starting lineup

> Draw the correct amount and concentration of the drug, and insert it into the PCA pump.

> Program the pump according to the manufacturer's direction

> Carefully read the PCA log, and then record the information based on your facility's policy.

Hit or miss

1. True.
2. False. You do need to note the number of times the patien received the I.V. drug throughout the time covered by you assessment (usually 4 hours).
3. True.
4. True.
5. True.

Page 155

trikeout

2. ~~It isn't necessary for each nurse who checks the PCA log to double-check the amount of fluid and drug in the syringe.~~ It's necessary for each nurse to do this.

atter's box

1. B, 2. A, 3. J, 4. I, 5. D, 6. H, 7. F, 8. G, 9. C, 10. E

Page 156

Match point

1. B, 2. C, 3. A

it or miss

1. True.
2. False. Heparin or insulin may be ordered in milliliters or units per hour, not per minute.
3. True.
4. False. Heparin prevents, not hastens, the formation of new clots and slows, not hastens, the development of pre-existing clots.
5. True.
6. True.

■ Page 157

Batter's box

1. F, 2. D, 3. B, 4. C, 5. E, 6. A

Dosage drills

Convert minutes to hours

60 min : 1 hour :: 1 min : X hour

60 min $\times$ X hour = 1 hour $\times$ 1 min

$$\frac{60 \text{ min} \times X \text{ hour}}{60 \text{ min}} = \frac{1 \text{ hour} \times 1 \text{ min}}{60 \text{ min}}$$

$X = \frac{1}{60}$

$X = 0.0166$ hr

Convert grams to milligrams

1 g = 1,000 mg

Change milligrams to milliliters

1,000 mg : 250 ml :: 2 mg : X ml

1,000 mg $\times$ X ml = 250 ml $\times$ 2 mg

$$\frac{1,000 \text{ mg} \times X \text{ ml}}{1,000 \text{ mg}} = \frac{250 \text{ mg} \times 1 \text{ mg}}{1,000 \text{ mg}}$$

$X = \frac{500}{1,000}$

$X = 0.5$ ml

Calculate the infusion rate

0.0166 hr : 0.5 ml :: 1 hr : X ml

0.0166 hr $\times$ X = 0.5 ml $\times$ 1 hr

$$\frac{0.0166 \text{ hr} \times X}{0.0166 \text{ hr}} = \frac{0.5 \text{ ml} \times 1 \text{ hr}}{0.0166 \text{ hr}}$$

$X = \frac{0.5}{0.0166}$

$X = 30.1$ or 30 ml/hr

■ Page 158

Starting lineup

$$\frac{25,000 \text{ units}}{1,000 \text{ ml}}$$

$$\frac{800 \text{ units/hour}}{X}$$

$$\frac{25,000 \text{ units}}{1,000 \text{ ml}} = \frac{800 \text{ units/hour}}{X}$$

$$25,000 \text{ units} \times X = 800 \text{ units/hour} \times 1,000 \text{ ml}$$

$$\frac{25,000 \text{ units} \times X}{25,000 \text{ units}} = \frac{800 \text{ units/hour} \times 1,000 \text{ ml}}{25,000 \text{ units}}$$

$$X = \frac{800,000 \text{ ml/hour}}{25,000}$$

$$X = 32 \text{ ml/hour}$$

■ Page 159

Dosage drills

Change minutes to hours

60 minutes : 1 hour : : 20 minutes : X hour

60 minutes $\times$ X hour = 1 hour $\times$ 20 minutes

$$\frac{60 \text{ minutes} \times X \text{ hour}}{60 \text{ minutes}} = \frac{1 \text{ hour} \times 20 \text{ minutes}}{60 \text{ minutes}}$$

$$X = \frac{20}{60}$$

X = 0.33 hour

Calculate the infusion rate

0.33 hr : 20 ml : : 1 hr : X ml

0.33 hr $\times$ X = 20 $\times$ 1 hr

$$\frac{0.33 \text{ hr} \times X}{0.33 \text{ hr}} = \frac{20 \text{ ml} \times 1 \text{ hr}}{0.33 \text{ hr}}$$

$$X = \frac{20}{0.03}$$

X = 60 ml/hr

Match point

1. B, 2. C, 3. A, 4. D, 5. E

■ Page 160

Starting lineup

$$\frac{10,000 \text{ units}}{250 \text{ ml}}$$

$$\frac{X}{30 \text{ ml/hour}}$$

$$\frac{10,000 \text{ units}}{250 \text{ ml}} = \frac{X}{30 \text{ ml/hour}}$$

$$250 \text{ ml} \times X = 30 \text{ ml/hour} \times 10,000 \text{ units}$$

$$\frac{250 \text{ ml} \times X}{250 \text{ ml}} = \frac{30 \text{ ml/hour} \times 10,000 \text{ units}}{250 \text{ ml}}$$

$$X = \frac{30 \times 10,000 \text{ units/hour}}{250}$$

$$X = \frac{300,000 \text{ units/hour}}{250}$$

$$X = 1,200 \text{ units/hour}$$

■ Page 161

Hit or miss

1. True.
2. True.
3. False. Regular insulin is the only insulin type that can be administered this way because it has a shorter duration of action than other insulins.
4. True.
5. False. An insulin infusion should be in a concentration of 1 unit/ml.

Batter's box

1. B, 2. F, 3. E, 4. D, 5. C, 6. A

■ Page 162

Dosage drills

Convert minutes to hours

$$0 \text{ min} : 1 \text{ hour} :: 1 \text{ min} : X \text{ hour}$$

$$0 \text{ min} \times X \text{ hour} = 1 \text{ hour} \times 1 \text{ min}$$

$$\frac{0 \text{ min} \times X \text{ hour}}{60 \text{ min}} = \frac{1 \text{ hour} \times 1 \text{ min}}{60 \text{ min}}$$

$$= \frac{1}{60}$$

$$= 0.0166 \text{ hr}$$

Change drops to milliliters

$$0 \text{ gtt} : 1 \text{ ml} :: 62 \text{ gtt} : X \text{ ml}$$

$$0 \text{ gtt} \times X \text{ ml} = 1 \text{ mg} \times 62 \text{ gtt}$$

$$\frac{0 \text{ gtt} \times X \text{ ml}}{60 \text{ gtt}} = \frac{1 \text{ mg} \times 62 \text{ gtt}}{60 \text{ gtt}}$$

$$= \frac{62}{60}$$

$$= 1.03 \text{ ml}$$

Calculate the infusion rate

$$0.0166 \text{ hr} : 1.03 \text{ ml} :: 1 \text{ hr} : X \text{ ml}$$

$$0.0166 \text{ hr} \times X = 1.03 \text{ ml} \times 1 \text{ hr}$$

$$\frac{0.0166 \text{ hr} \times X}{0.0166 \text{ hr}} = \frac{1.03 \text{ ml} \times 1 \text{ hr}}{0.0166 \text{ hr}}$$

$$= \frac{1.03}{0.0166 \text{ hr}}$$

$$= 62.04 \text{ or } 62 \text{ ml/hr}$$

Calculate the amount infused

$$= 62 \text{ ml/hr} \times 4 \text{ hr}$$

$$= 248 \text{ ml}$$

Starting lineup

100 units: 100 ml

X : 5 ml/hour

100 units: 100 ml :: X : 5 ml/hour

$X \times 100 \text{ ml}/100 \text{ ml} = 100 \text{ units} \times 5 \text{ ml/hour}$

$\dfrac{X \times 100 \text{ ml}}{100 \text{ ml}} = \dfrac{100 \text{ units} \times 5 \text{ ml/hour}}{100 \text{ ml}}$

$X = 5$ units/hour

■ Page 163

Hit or miss

1. True.
2. True.
3. False. Electrolytes can be given in small-volume, intermittent infusions piggybacked into existing I.V. lines, not administered I.M.
4. False. This is sometimes necessary.
5. True.

Strikeout

3. ~~To calculate the amount of additive, use the fraction method.~~ To calculate the amount of additive, you should use the proportion method as you would for any prepared liquid drug.

■ Page 164

Starting lineup

50 mg: 1 ml

75 mg : X

50 mg : 1 ml :: 75 mg : X

$X \times 50 \text{ mg} = 75 \text{ mg} \times 1 \text{ ml}$

$\dfrac{X \times 50 \text{ mg}}{50 \text{ mg}} = \dfrac{75 \text{ mg} \times 1 \text{ ml}}{50 \text{ mg}}$

$X = \dfrac{75 \text{ ml}}{50}$

$X = 1.5$ ml

$\dfrac{1{,}000 \text{ ml}}{12 \text{ hr}} = 83.3 \text{ ml/hr}$

Batter's box

1. E, 2. A, 3. F, 4. B, 5. C, 6. D

■ Page 165

Starting lineup

500 mg : 5 ml

250 mg : X

500 mg : 5 ml :: 250 mg : X

500 mg × X = 250 mg × 5 ml

$\dfrac{\cancel{500\ mg} \times X}{\cancel{500\ mg}} = \dfrac{250\ \cancel{mg} \times 5\ ml}{500\ \cancel{mg}}$

$X = \dfrac{250 \times 5\ ml}{500}$

$X = \dfrac{1{,}250\ ml}{500}$

$X = 2.5\ ml$

Hit or miss

Answer: True.

■ Page 166

Strikeout

2. ~~After calculating an I.V. piggyback dose, it isn't necessary to make sure that the drugs mixed in the same syringe or I.V. bag are compatible.~~ This is a necessary step after calculating an I.V. piggyback dose.

Dosage drills

1 hour = 60 minutes

Change milliliters to drops

1 ml : 15 gtt : : 250 ml : X gtt

1 ml × X gtt = 15 gtt × 250 ml

$\dfrac{\cancel{1\ ml} \times X\ gtt}{\cancel{1\ ml}} = \dfrac{15\ gtt \times 250\ \cancel{ml}}{1\ \cancel{ml}}$

$X = 3{,}750$ gtt

Calculate the flow rate

60 min : 3,750 gtt : : 1 min : X gtt

60 min × X gtt = 3,750 gtt × 1 min

$\dfrac{\cancel{60\ min} \times X\ gtt}{\cancel{60\ min}} = \dfrac{3{,}750\ gtt \times 1\ \cancel{min}}{60\ \cancel{min}}$

$X = \dfrac{3{,}750}{60}$

$X = 62.5$ gtt/min

■ Page 167

Batter's box

1. C, 2. D, 3. E, 4. B, 5. A

Hit or miss

1. True.
2. False. A catheter smaller than 18G is used for elderly and pediatric patients.
3. True.
4. False. A unit of whole blood or packed red blood cells should infuse for no longer than 4, not 6, hours because the blood can deteriorate and become contaminated after this time.

Page 168

osage drills

$$\text{hr} : 250 \text{ ml} :: 1 \text{ hr} : X \text{ ml}$$

$$\text{hr} \times X \text{ ml} = 250 \text{ ml} \times 1 \text{ hr}$$

$$\frac{\cancel{\text{hr}} \times X \text{ ml}}{4 \cancel{\text{hr}}} = \frac{250 \text{ ml} \times 1 \cancel{\text{hr}}}{4 \cancel{\text{hr}}}$$

$$= \frac{250}{4}$$

$$= 62.5 \text{ or } 63 \text{ ml/hr}$$

atter's box

1. C, 2. A, 3. B, 4. E, 5. D

Page 169

tarting lineup

Find the flow rate in milliliters per minute.

Multiply the flow rate by the drop factor to find the drip rate in drops per minute.

atter's box

D, 2. E, 3. F, 4. C, 5. A, 6. B

■ Page 170

Hit or miss

1. True.
2. False. After TPN is infused at a slow initial rate, it's gradually, not rapidly, increased to a maintenance level.
3. True.
4. False. To set the maintenance flow rate of a TPN infusion pump, you must find the flow rate per hour, not per minute.
5. True.

Dosage drills

$$25,000 \text{ units} : 250 \text{ ml} :: 1,400 \text{ units} \times X \text{ ml}$$

$$25,000 \text{ units} \times X \text{ ml} = 250 \text{ ml} \times 1,400 \text{ units}$$

$$\frac{25,000 \cancel{\text{units}} \times X \text{ ml}}{25,000 \cancel{\text{units}}} = \frac{250 \text{ ml} \times 1,400 \cancel{\text{units}}}{25,000 \cancel{\text{units}}}$$

$$X = \frac{350,000}{25,000}$$

$$X = 14 \text{ ml/hr}$$

■ Page 171

Starting lineup

$\dfrac{22.5 \text{ ml}}{60 \text{ minutes}}$

$X = \dfrac{22.5 \cancel{\text{ml}}}{60 \text{ minutes}} \times \dfrac{20 \text{ gtt}}{\cancel{\text{ml}}}$

$X = \dfrac{22.5 \times 20 \text{ gtt}}{60 \text{ minutes}}$

$X = \dfrac{450 \text{ gtt}}{60 \text{ minutes}}$

$X = 7.5 \text{ gtt/minute}$

Dosage drills

$$1 \text{ hr} : 40 \text{ ml} :: 8 \text{ hr} : X \text{ ml}$$

$$1 \text{ hr} \times X \text{ ml} = 40 \text{ ml} \times 8 \text{ hr}$$

$$\frac{1 \cancel{\text{hr}} \times X \text{ ml}}{1 \cancel{\text{hr}}} = \frac{40 \text{ ml} \times 8 \cancel{\text{hr}}}{1 \cancel{\text{hr}}}$$

$$X = 40 \times 8$$

$$X = 320 \text{ ml}$$

■ Page 172

Dosage drills

100 ml : 400 mg :: 2 ml : X mg

100 ml × X mg = 400 mg × 2 ml

$$\frac{\cancel{100\ ml} \times X\,mg}{\cancel{100\ ml}} = \frac{400\,mg \times 2\,\cancel{ml}}{100\,\cancel{ml}}$$

$$X = \frac{800}{100}$$

X = 8 mg/hr

Starting lineup

$$X = \frac{750\ ml}{(50\ gtt/minute \div 10\ gtt/ml) \div 60\ min}$$

$$\frac{50\ \cancel{gtt}}{1\ min} \times \frac{1\ ml}{10\ \cancel{gtt}} = \frac{5\ ml}{minute}$$

$$X = \frac{750\ \cancel{ml}}{\dfrac{5\ \cancel{ml}}{1\ \cancel{min}} \times \dfrac{60\ \cancel{min}}{1\ hour}}$$

$$X = \frac{750}{5 \times 60\ hours}$$

$$X = \frac{750}{300\ hours}$$

$$X = 2.5\ hours$$

■ Chapter 7

■ Page 176

Strikeout

1. ~~Drug administration for children is the same as it is for adults.~~ The pharmacokinetics, pharmacodynamics, and pharmacotherapeutics of drugs differ greatly between children and adults.
2. ~~Children receive drugs via different routes than adults do.~~ Both children and adults receive drugs via the oral, subcutaneous, intramuscular, I.V., and topical routes.
5. ~~An incorrect drug dose is more likely to harm an adult than a child.~~ An incorrect dose is more likely to harm a child than an adult.
7. ~~When a liquid form of the drug isn't available, you should crush the tablet or capsule and put it in breast milk or infant formula.~~ You shouldn't use essential fluids, such as breast milk or infant formula, because this could lead to feeding refusal.

■ Page 177

Match point

1. C, 2. E, 3. A, 4. B, 5. D

Hit or miss

1. True.
2. False. If you're unsure of the correct dosage, consult a formulary or drug handbook. When in doubt, call the pharmacist.
3. True.

■ Page 178

Starting lineup

$$\frac{20\ mg}{1\ kg/dose} = \frac{X}{9\ kg/dose}$$

$$X \times 1\ kg/dose = 20\ mg \times 9\ kg/dose$$

$$\frac{X \times \cancel{1\ kg/dose}}{1\ kg/dose} = \frac{20\ mg \times 9\ \cancel{kg/dose}}{1\ \cancel{kg/dose}}$$

$$X = 180\ mg$$

Dosage drills

2.2 lb : 1 kg :: 32 lb : X kg

2.2 lb × X kg = 1 kg × 32 lb

$$\frac{\cancel{2.2\ lb} \times X\,kg}{2.2\ \cancel{lb}} = \frac{1\ kg \times 32\ \cancel{lb}}{2.2\ \cancel{lb}}$$

$$X = \frac{32}{2.2}$$

X = 14.5454 kg

1 kg: 25 mg :: 14.5454 kg : X mg

1 kg × X mg = 25 mg × 14.5454 kg

$$\frac{\cancel{1\ kg} \times X\,mg}{1\ \cancel{kg}} = \frac{25\,mg \times 14.5454\ \cancel{kg}}{1\ \cancel{kg}}$$

X = 25 × 14.5454

X = 363.6 mg

■ Page 179

Match point

1. D, 2. B, 3. F, 4. I, 5. G, 6. A, 7. E, 8. C, 9. H

Page 180

Batter's box

1. A, 2. C, 3. B

Dosage drills

L = 1,000 ml

$000\ ml : 8\ g :: 25\ ml : X\ g$

$000\ ml \times X\ g = 125\ ml \times 8\ g$

$$\frac{000\ ml \times X\ g}{1{,}000\ ml} = \frac{125\ ml \times 8\ g}{1{,}000\ ml}$$

$$= \frac{1{,}000}{1{,}000}$$

$$= 1\ g/hr$$

Page 181

Match point

1. C, 2. A, 3. B

Page 182

Batter's box

1. D or C, 2. C or D, 3. A, 4. B

Dosage drills

$1\ kg : 15\ mg :: 20\ kg : X\ mg$

$1\ kg \times X\ mg = 15\ mg \times 20\ kg$

$$\frac{1\ kg \times X\ mg}{1\ kg} = \frac{15\ mg \times 20\ kg}{1\ kg}$$

$X = 15 \times 20$

$X = 300\ mg$

Page 183

Starting lineup

Use the nomogram to determine that
the child's BSA is 0.66 m².

Set up an equation using the appropriate formula.
Divide the child's BSA by 1.73 m² (the average adult BSA),
and multiply by the average adult dose, 1,000 mg:

$$X = \frac{0.66\ m^2}{1.73\ m^2} \times 1{,}000\ mg$$

Solve for X by canceling units that appear in both the
numerator and denominator, multiplying the child's BSA
by the average adult dose, and dividing the result
by the average adult BSA:

$$X = \frac{0.66\ m^2 \times 1{,}000\ mg}{1.73\ m^2}$$

$$X = 381.5\ mg$$

Match point

1. C, 2. D, 3. A, 4. B

■ Pages 184 and 185

A-maze-ing race

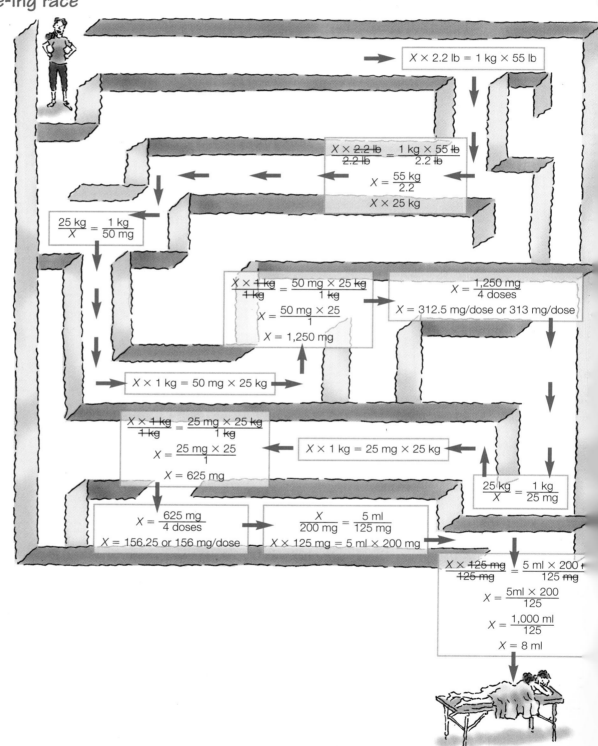

$X \times 2.2 \text{ lb} = 1 \text{ kg} \times 55 \text{ lb}$

$\dfrac{X \times \cancel{2.2 \text{ lb}}}{2.2 \text{ lb}} = \dfrac{1 \text{ kg} \times 55 \cancel{\text{lb}}}{2.2 \text{ lb}}$

$X = \dfrac{55 \text{ kg}}{2.2}$

$X \times 25 \text{ kg}$

$\dfrac{25 \text{ kg}}{X} = \dfrac{1 \text{ kg}}{50 \text{ mg}}$

$\dfrac{X \times \cancel{1 \text{ kg}}}{1 \text{ kg}} = \dfrac{50 \text{ mg} \times 25 \cancel{\text{kg}}}{1 \text{ kg}}$

$X = \dfrac{50 \text{ mg} \times 25}{1}$

$X = 1{,}250 \text{ mg}$

$X = \dfrac{1{,}250 \text{ mg}}{4 \text{ doses}}$

$X = 312.5 \text{ mg/dose or } 313 \text{ mg/dose}$

$X \times 1 \text{ kg} = 50 \text{ mg} \times 25 \text{ kg}$

$\dfrac{X \times \cancel{1 \text{ kg}}}{1 \text{ kg}} = \dfrac{25 \text{ mg} \times 25 \cancel{\text{kg}}}{1 \text{ kg}}$

$X = \dfrac{25 \text{ mg} \times 25}{1}$

$X = 625 \text{ mg}$

$X \times 1 \text{ kg} = 25 \text{ mg} \times 25 \text{ kg}$

$\dfrac{25 \text{ kg}}{X} = \dfrac{1 \text{ kg}}{25 \text{ mg}}$

$X = \dfrac{625 \text{ mg}}{4 \text{ doses}}$

$X = 156.25 \text{ or } 156 \text{ mg/dose}$

$\dfrac{X}{200 \text{ mg}} = \dfrac{5 \text{ ml}}{125 \text{ mg}}$

$X \times 125 \text{ mg} = 5 \text{ ml} \times 200 \text{ mg}$

$\dfrac{X \times \cancel{125 \text{ mg}}}{125 \text{ mg}} = \dfrac{5 \text{ ml} \times 200 +}{125 \text{ mg}}$

$X = \dfrac{5 \text{ ml} \times 200}{125}$

$X = \dfrac{1{,}000 \text{ ml}}{125}$

$X = 8 \text{ ml}$

Page 186

Starting lineup

Calculate the dosage.

Draw up the drug in a syringe, then add the drug to the I.V. bag or fluid chamber through the drug additive port, using aseptic technique.

Mix the drug thoroughly.

Label the I.V. bag or fluid chamber with the drug's name, the dosage, the time and date it was mixed, and your initials.

Hang the solution and administer the drug by infusion pump at the prescribed flow rate.

Page 187

Jumble gym

. Volume-control devices are calibrated in 1-ml increments.
. Intermittent infusion is used commonly in acute and home care settings.
. Medication-filled syringes with microtubing can be used to infuse small volumes via syringe pumps.
. Accuracy is especially important with pediatric patients.

Answer: Absorption

Starting lineup

Carefully calculate the prescribed volume of drug.

Draw up the prescribed volume of drug into the syringe.

Add the drug to the fluid chamber through the drug additive port.

Mix the drug thoroughly.

Label the volume-control device with the name of the drug.

Attach the volume-control device to an electronic infusion pump to control the infusion rate.

Calculate the appropriate flow rate and infuse the drug.

Flush the line to clear the tubing of the drug.

Disconnect the device when the flush is complete.

Page 188

Dosage drills

$1.73 \text{ m}^2 : 60 \text{ mg} :: 0.55 \text{ m}^2 : X \text{ mg}$

$1.73 \text{ m}^2 \times X \text{ mg} = 60 \text{ mg} \times 0.55 \text{ m}^2$

$$\frac{\cancel{1.73 \text{ m}^2} \times X \text{ mg}}{\cancel{1.73 \text{ m}^2}} = \frac{60 \text{ mg} \times 0.55 \cancel{\text{m}^2}}{1.73 \cancel{\text{m}^2}}$$

$X = \dfrac{33}{1.73}$

$X = 19.1 \text{ mg}$

Page 189

Strikeout

$$\frac{\cancel{24 \text{ lb}}}{\cancel{X}} = \frac{\cancel{100 \text{ kcal}}}{\cancel{1100 \text{ kcal}}}$$

In this case, setting up a proportion that includes the patient's weight isn't relevant because you're calculating fluid needs based on calories, not body surface area.

Batter's box

1. C, 2. B, 3. A

Page 190

Match point

1. A, 2. C, 3. B, 4. D

Hit or miss

1. False. BSA is determined through the intersection of height and weight on a nomogram.
2. False. To calculate the daily fluid needs of a child who isn't dehydrated, you should multiply the BSA by 1,500, not 1,100.
3. True.
4. True.

■ Page 191

Dosage drills

1. First, calculate the required milligrams:

1 kg : 5 mg :: 23.6 kg : X mg

1 kg × X mg = 5 mg × 23.6 kg

$$\frac{\cancel{1\ kg} \times X\ mg}{\cancel{1\ kg}} = \frac{5\ mg \times 23.6\ \cancel{kg}}{1\ \cancel{kg}}$$

X = 118 mg

2. Then calculate the required milliliters:

125 mg : 5 ml :: 118 mg : X ml

125 mg × X ml = 5 ml × 118 mg

$$\frac{\cancel{125\ mg} \times X\ ml}{\cancel{125\ mg}} = \frac{5\ ml \times 118\ \cancel{mg}}{125\ \cancel{mg}}$$

X = $\frac{590}{125}$

X = 4.7 ml

3. Finally, determine the amount per dose:

4.7 ml : 2 doses :: X ml : 1 dose

4.7 ml × 1 dose = 2 doses × X ml

$$\frac{4.7\ ml \times 1\ \cancel{dose}}{2\ \cancel{doses}} = \frac{2\ \cancel{doses} \times X\ ml}{2\ \cancel{doses}}$$

X = $\frac{4.7}{2}$

X = 2.35 ml/dose

Match point

1. C, 2. A, 3. B

■ Page 192

Cross-training

				¹L	I	Q	U	²I	D		³C			
								N			A			
			⁴B	U	R	E	T	R	O	L				
				E				R		O		⁵B		
		⁶I					R	⁷C	R	U	S	H		
⁸N	O	M	O	⁹G	R	A	M			I		A		
			R				I			E				
			E				T		¹⁰S	U	B	Q		
	¹¹F		A				T		E					
	L		T				E							
¹²D	I	L	U	T	E	D	N							
			I				R							
			D				T							

■ Page 193

Strikeout

2. ~~To improve renal function~~
3. ~~To minimize maternal weight gain~~
5. ~~To support fetal growth~~

Batter's box

1. D, 2. A, 3. E, 4. F, 5. B, 6. C

■ Page 194

Hit or miss

1. True.
2. False. This statement applies to magnesium sulfate, not to dinoprostone.
3. True.
4. False. This statement applies to oxytocin, not to magnesium sulfate.
5. True.
6. True.

Jumble gym

1. Magnesium sulfate prevents or controls seizures that may be caused by gestational hypertension.
2. Dinoprostone is available as an endocervical gel or a vaginal insert or suppository.
3. After labor is established, the doctor may decrease the infusion rate of oxytocin.
4. When administering dinoprostone, have the patient lie on her back.

Answer: Placenta

■ Page 195

Match point

1. C, 2. A, 3. B

Page 196

Dosage drills

First, find the strength of the solution:

: 250 ml :: X mg : 1 ml

$X \times 250$ ml = 10 mg $\times$ 1 ml

$\dfrac{X \times 250\ \text{ml}}{50\ \text{ml}} = \dfrac{10\ \text{mg} \times 1\ \text{ml}}{250\ \text{ml}}$

$\dfrac{0}{50}$

04 mg

Then, convert to micrograms by multiplying by 1,000:

40 mcg :: X ml : 5 mcg

$X \times 40$ mcg = 1 ml $\times$ 5 mcg

$\dfrac{X \times 40\ \text{mcg}}{40\ \text{mcg}} = \dfrac{1\ \text{ml} \times 5\ \text{mcg}}{40\ \text{mcg}}$

$\dfrac{5}{0}$

.125 ml/minute

ml : 1 minute = X ml : 60 minutes

$\dfrac{X \times 1\ \text{minute}}{\text{minute}} = \dfrac{0.125\ \text{ml} \times 60\ \text{minutes}}{1\ \text{minute}}$

.125 $\times$ 60

.5 ml/hour

Starting lineup

Calculate the strength of the solution by setting up a proportion with the known strength in one fraction and the unknown strength in the other fraction.

Cross-multiply the fractions.

Solve for X by dividing each side of the equation by 500 ml.

Calculate the flow rate by setting up another proportion with the solution concentration in one fraction and the unknown flow rate the other fraction. Cross-multiply the fractions and solve for X.

■ Page 197

Cross-training

■ Page 198

Train your brain

Answer: Proportions can be used to solve obstetric dosage calculations.

Jumble gym

1. Many I.V. drugs are administered in life-threatening situations.
2. On a critical care unit, you need to perform dosage calculations quickly.
3. The nurse's job is to prepare the drug for infusion, give it to the patient, and then observe him to evaluate the drug's effectiveness.

Answer: I.V. push

■ Page 199

Match point

1. B, 2. A, 3. C

■ Page 200

Dosage drills

73 kg : X mcg/minute : : 1 kg : 50 mcg/minute

73 kg × 50 mcg/minute = 1 kg × X mcg/minute

$$\frac{73 \ \cancel{kg} \times 50 \ \text{mcg/minute}}{1 \ \cancel{kg}} = \frac{\cancel{1 \ kg} \times X \ \text{mcg/minute}}{\cancel{1 \ kg}}$$

X = 3,650 mcg/minute

3.65 mg : X ml = 2,500 mg : 250 ml

3.650 mg × 250 ml = X ml × 2,500 mg

$$\frac{3.650 \ \cancel{mg} \times 250 \ \text{ml}}{2,500 \ \cancel{mg}} = \frac{X \ \text{ml} \times \cancel{2,500 \ mg}}{\cancel{2,500 \ mg}}$$

$X = \dfrac{912.5}{2,500}$

X = 0.365 ml/minute

0.365 ml/minute × 60 minutes/hr = 21.9 or 22 ml/hour

Match point

1. C, 2. B, 3. C, 4. B, 5. A, 6. C, 7. A

■ Page 201

Batter's box

1. B, 2. C, 3. A

Hit or miss

1. True.
2. False. You should multiply by the drug's concentration.
3. False. You should multiply by 1,000, not 100.

■ Page 202

Dosage drills

106 kg : X mcg/minute : : 1 kg : 5 mcg/minute

106 kg × 5 mcg/minute = 1 kg × X mcg/minute

$$\frac{106 \ \cancel{kg} \times 5 \ \text{mcg/minute}}{1 \ \cancel{kg}} = \frac{\cancel{1 \ kg} \times X \ \text{mcg/minute}}{\cancel{1 \ kg}}$$

X = 530 mcg/minute

0.530 mg : X ml = 500 mg : 250 ml

0.530 mg × 250 ml = X ml × 500 mg

$$\frac{0.530 \ \cancel{mg} \times 250 \ \text{ml}}{2,500 \ \cancel{mg}} = \frac{X \ \text{ml} \times \cancel{500 \ mg}}{\cancel{500 \ mg}}$$

$X = \dfrac{132.5}{500}$

X = 0.265 ml/minute

■ Page 203

Match point

1. C, 2. A, 3. B

Dosage drills

$\dfrac{20 \ \text{mg}}{200 \ \text{ml}} \times 1,000 = 100 \ \text{mcg/ml}$

$\dfrac{100 \ \text{mcg/ml}}{60 \ \text{minutes}} = 1.667 \ \text{mcg/ml/minute}$

$\dfrac{1.667 \ \text{mcg/ml/minute}}{90 \ \text{kg}} = 0.0185 \ \text{mcg/kg/ml/minute} \times 20 \ \text{ml}$

Dose = 0.37 mcg/kg/minute

Page 204

Batter's box

1. C, 2. B, 3. A

Starting lineup

$$X = \frac{200 \text{ mg}}{500 \text{ ml}}$$

$$X = 0.4 \text{ mg/ml}$$

$$0.4 \text{ mg/ml} \times 1,000 = 400 \text{ mcg/ml}$$

$$\frac{25 \text{ mcg/minute}}{X \text{ ml/minute}} = \frac{400 \text{ mcg}}{1 \text{ ml}}$$

$$X \text{ ml/minute} \times 400 \text{ mcg} = 25 \text{ mcg/minute} \times 1 \text{ ml}$$

$$\frac{X \text{ ml/minute} \times \cancel{400 \text{ mcg}}}{\cancel{400 \text{ mcg}}} = \frac{25 \cancel{\text{mcg}}/\text{minute} \times 1 \text{ ml}}{400 \cancel{\text{mcg}}}$$

$$X = \frac{25 \text{ ml/minute}}{400}$$

$$X = 0.0625 \text{ ml/minute}$$

■ Page 205

Dosage drills

$$4 \text{ mg} : 250 \text{ ml} :: X \text{ mg} : 1 \text{ ml}$$

$$X \text{ mg} \times 250 \text{ ml} = 1 \text{ ml} \times 4 \text{ mg}$$

$$\frac{X \text{ mg} \times \cancel{250 \text{ ml}}}{\cancel{250 \text{ ml}}} = \frac{1 \cancel{\text{ml}} \times 4 \text{ mg}}{250 \cancel{\text{ml}}}$$

$$X = \frac{4 \text{ mg}}{250}$$

$$X = 0.016 \text{ mg/ml}$$

$$X = 16 \text{ mcg/ml}$$

$$30 \text{ ml} : 60 \text{ minutes} :: X \text{ ml} : 1 \text{ minute}$$

$$30 \text{ ml} \times 1 \text{ minute} = 60 \text{ minutes} \times X \text{ ml}$$

$$\frac{30 \text{ ml} \times 1 \cancel{\text{minute}}}{60 \cancel{\text{minutes}}} = \frac{\cancel{60 \text{ minutes}} \times X \text{ ml}}{\cancel{60 \text{ minutes}}}$$

$$X = \frac{30}{60}$$

$$X = 0.5 \text{ ml/minute}$$

$$X = 0.5 \text{ ml/minute} \times 16 \text{ mcg/ml}$$

$$X = 8 \text{ mcg/minute}$$

Strikeout

$$\cancel{X \times 2.2 \text{ lb} = 1 \text{ kg} \times 70 \text{ ml}}$$

In this equation, you're calculating the patient's weight in kilograms, so 1 kg should be multiplied by the patient's weight (200 lb), not by 70 ml.

Notes

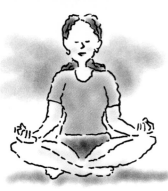

Notes

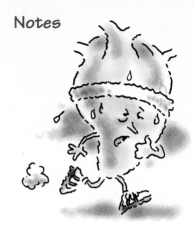

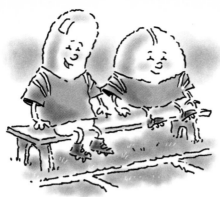

Notes

Notes

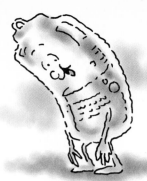

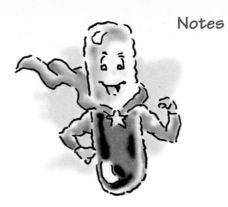

Notes

Notes

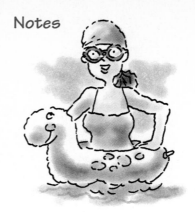

Notes

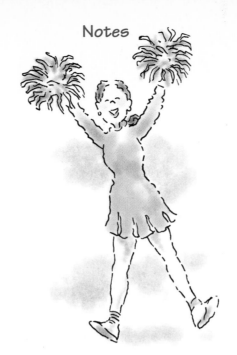